Overcoming Anxiety, Stress and Panic

A Five Areas Approach

Second Edition

Dr Chris Williams MBChB BSc MMedSc MD FRCPsych BABCP Accredited CBT practitioner
Professor of Psychosocial Psychiatry and Honorary Consultant Psychiatrist,
Section of Psychological Medicine,
Faculty of Medicine,
University of Glasgow, UK

Helping you to help yourself
www.livinglifetothefull.com
www.fiveareas.com

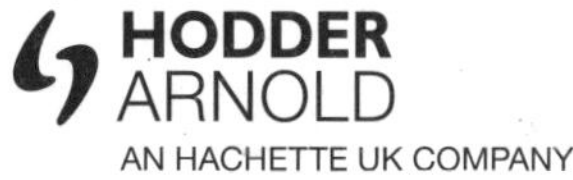

First published in Great Britain in 2010 by
Hodder Arnold, an imprint of Hodder Education,
an Hachette UK company, 338 Euston Road, London NW1 3BH

http://www.hodderarnold.com

British Library Cataloguing in Publication Data
A catalogue record for this book is available from the British Library

Library of Congress Cataloging-in-Publication Data
A catalog record for this book is available from the Library of Congress

ISBN-13 978-0-340-98655-4

2 3 4 5 6 7 8 9 10

Commissioning Editor: Caroline Makepeace
Project Editor: Francesca Naish
Production Controller: Kate Harris
Cover Design: Lynda King

Typeset in 11pt Frutiger by Pantek Arts Ltd., Maidstone, Kent.
Printed and bound in Malta.

What do you think about this book? Or any other Hodder Arnold title?

Please visit our website: **www.hodderarnold.com**
Or email us at **admin@fiveareas.com**

Please visit the Five Areas website (**www.fiveareas.com**) for more information about the range of Five Areas resources.

New ways of accessing the workbooks

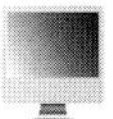

Electronic (PDF) versions of the workbooks are available from the publisher for restricted access on password-protected health service computer servers to allow high-quality copies of the workbooks to be printed off by a defined number of practitioners.

For more information please contact: Jenny Davis, Rights Manager, Hodder Education, 338 Euston Road, London NW1 3BH.
Tel: +44 (0) 20 7873 6286, email: **jenny.davis@hodder.co.uk**

Buying the books in bulk: Bulk copies of the book are available at discounted rates direct from the publisher.

To take advantage of these reduced rates please contact: Jane MacRae, Sales Development Manager, Hodder Education, 338 Euston Road, London NW1 3BH.
Tel: +44 (0) 20 7873 6146, email: **jane.macrae@hodder.co.uk**

Translations and large print versions

For **translation requests** and **large print versions** please contact **admin@fiveareas.com**.

Contents

Two additional online workbooks, *Understanding and using anti-anxiety medication* and *Planning for the future* are available free from **www.livinglifetothefull.com**.

Introduction

Welcome to this second edition of *Overcoming Anxiety, Stress and Panic: A Five Areas Approach*. Problems of anxiety and depression are common difficulties that can affect anyone at some stage in their lives. Anxiety can affect people in many different ways – worry, stress, panic attacks and phobias – which are the focus of this book.

This book is designed to actively help you to:

- Learn important information about how anxiety, stress, panic or phobias can affect your life.
- Work out why you are feeling as you do.
- Learn and practise some practical skills to help change how you feel.

By following the clearly described tools in these workbooks, you can make helpful changes to your life.

Who are the workbooks for?

You may be using the workbooks for yourself, or perhaps you are a close friend or family member wanting to know more about anxiety and how to help. Many healthcare practitioners also use the workbooks in this series to support those they work with.

Self-help approaches can be used by people with problems ranging from mild distress through to more severe anxiety or depression. The key thing is that you feel **able** to use the materials and **want** to use this approach.

Using the workbooks

The course involves **reading** the course workbooks and also **working** on problems by putting into practice the things you are learning. Picking the right time to do the course is important. For example, if your concentration, energy or motivation levels are far lower than usual, you may find it very hard to keep your mind on things or to make changes. Other approaches may be more appropriate first – allowing you to come back to use the workbooks at a time when you are able to get the most from them. If you find that you are struggling to use the workbooks, or you feel worse as you work through them, please discuss this with your doctor or other healthcare practitioner. The course is not meant to replace getting the right level of support for more severe mental health problems.

Which workbook should you use first?

There is no right or wrong way to use the workbooks. Many people find it helpful to first read the workbooks in Part 1: *Tackling your anxiety: starting out (... and how to keep going if you feel stuck)*, then either *Understanding worry and stress* or *Understanding panic and phobias* depending on which most applies to your own situation.

These will give you a good overview of the approach and will also help you to decide which of the *Making changes* workbooks in Part 2 of the book you should read. You can use as many or as few workbooks in the course as you wish. You will feel most motivated to try to make changes if you use the workbooks that tackle problems you have noticed in your life and that you want to change.

Key point

The key to creating change in your life is **using** the workbooks and **putting what you learn into practice**.

Getting help from others

It can be hard making changes when you feel very stressed or low. Many people start off trying to improve things with lots of motivation. But part of feeling stressed is that you can sometimes quickly give up on change. That's entirely normal and is very human (think how hard people find it keeping New Year resolutions even when they aren't feeling worried about things).

Time and time again, people using resources like this have found the benefits of working with someone else to support and encourage them when things feel hard. We therefore suggest that you partner up with someone to help you as you use the course. For example, a health or social services worker, your doctor, a voluntary sector worker or a trusted family member or friend.

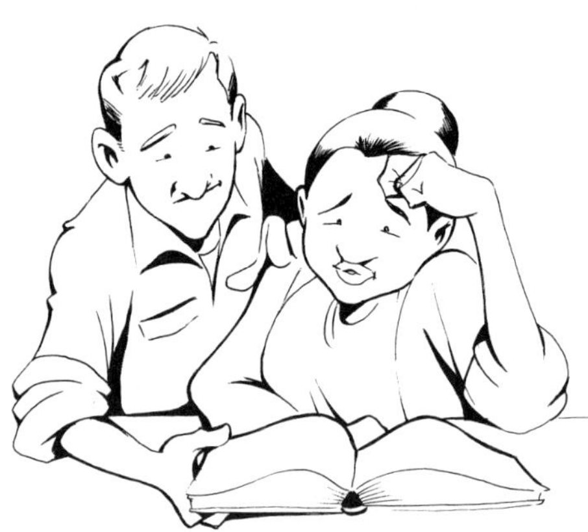

The important thing is to have someone else there, helping you, discussing problems that seem hard – and to say well done when things move forwards. If you aren't sure where to seek help from others, check out the last sections of the workbooks *Understanding worry and stress* and *Understanding panic and phobias*. You will find a list of useful support options you can look at if you find yourself struggling.

A word of encouragement

Anxiety, stress and panic affect many people at some time in their life. Fortunately, it has now become clear that by changing certain thoughts and behaviour patterns you can greatly improve how you feel. The content of these workbooks is based on the cognitive behavioural therapy (CBT; a kind of talking treatment) approach. The developers of CBT have found many effective ways of tackling the common symptoms and problems people face when feeling anxious.

This course is written in a way that clearly explains what to do, so that you can test the effect of these different suggestions in your own life. The workbooks aim to help you to **regain a sense of control** over how you feel.

The self-help approach can really work

Research has been done on people who use books like this one based on CBT. Treatment guidelines often recommend the use of CBT self-help approaches like this as a treatment for anxiety, panic and phobias. The course can make a big difference if you can commit to using it.

Making a commitment

Sometimes making changes is easier said (or written) than done. All of us feel discouraged and overwhelmed from time to time. This is even more likely when you feel distressed, anxious, tense or low.

Therefore, **try to make a commitment to use this course** and to keep at it even if you feel discouraged or stuck for some time. To do this you will need to **pace yourself** by using a step-by-step approach. Having someone else to encourage you is also important. The research on these approaches shows just how helpful this can be. Also, be realistic. Bear in mind your motivation and energy levels so that you don't try to do more than you can at one time. This will help you to get as much from the course as you can.

The *Tackling your anxiety: starting out (... and how to keep going if you feel stuck)* workbook gives some suggestions of how you can **pace things**, and also some suggestions of what to do if you are struggling.

New online resources

Two online resources are available to support users of the course:

1. **www.livinglifetothefull.com**. This free website contains short talks that help you to build upon the course workbooks. There is also a moderated chat room where people can swap ideas, hints and tips, as well as offering and receiving mutual support. If you don't have a computer, try to use one in an internet café, or in a public library. Sign up for the free reminder letters there to also help you keep on track. You can also freely access TV-based versions of the course from the website. Some people like to see and hear how other people have applied what they have learned. Again, using the site with support and encouragement from someone can be a big help to getting the most out of the approach.

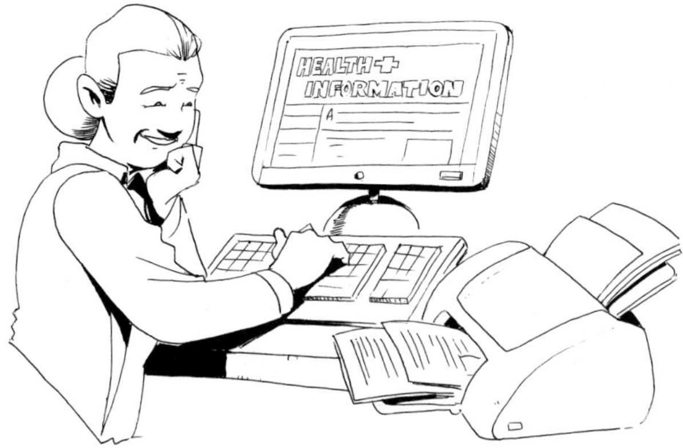

2. The **www.fiveareas.com** website also has a list of other Five Areas resources, including self-help books, free handouts and downloads (including MP3s of relaxation techniques) and more.

A note about copyright

Acknowledgements

The illustrations in the workbooks have been produced by Keith Chan, kchan75@hotmail.com. Copies are available as a separate download for clinical use at www.fiveareas.com.

Finally, I wish to thank Alison, Hannah and Andrew, who have supported me during the writing of this book

Dr Chris Williams
December 2009

PART 1

Understanding why you feel as you do

Overcoming Anxiety, Stress and Panic

A Five Areas Approach

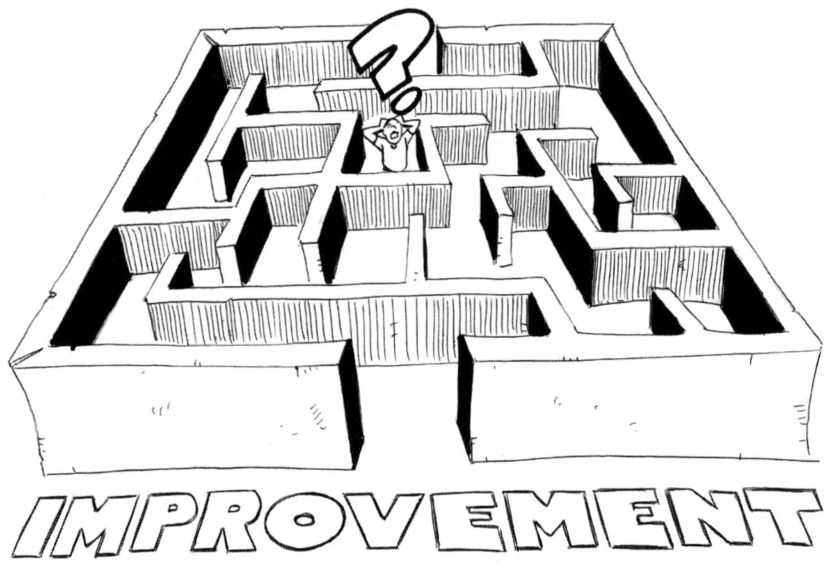

Tackling your anxiety: starting out (… and how to keep going if you feel stuck)

www.livinglifetothefull.com
www.fiveareas.com

Dr Chris Williams

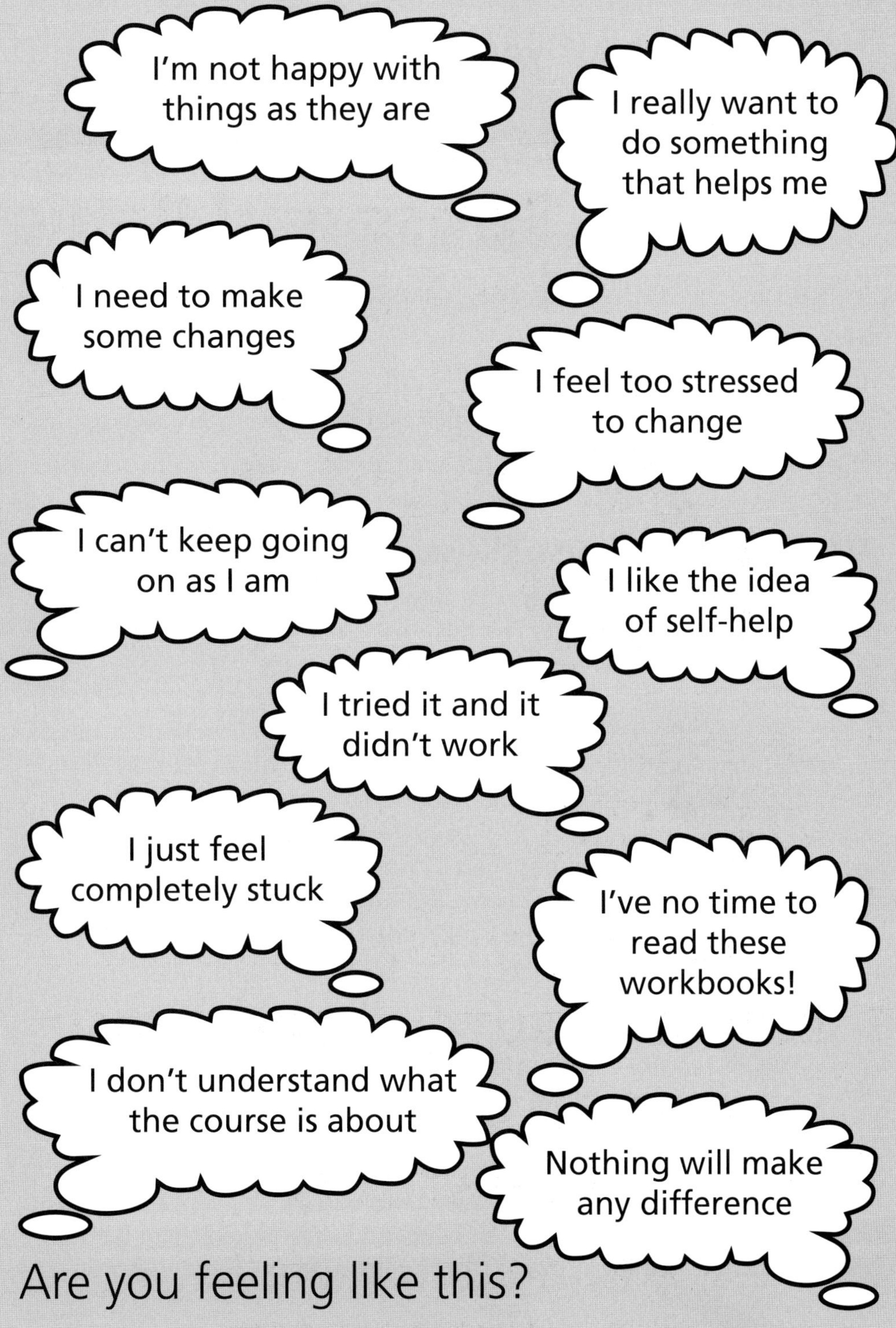
I'm not happy with things as they are
I really want to do something that helps me
I need to make some changes
I feel too stressed to change
I can't keep going on as I am
I like the idea of self-help
I tried it and it didn't work
I just feel completely stuck
I've no time to read these workbooks!
I don't understand what the course is about
Nothing will make any difference

Are you feeling like this?

If so … this **course is for you**.

In this workbook you will:

- Learn how to get the most out of this course.
- Make a clear but flexible plan of when to use this and the other workbooks.
- Discover how to overcome common blocks to change.

About the course

The workbooks in this course aim to help you understand why you feel as you do. They will teach you important life skills that will help you to turn the corner, and improve how you feel.

Why should you use these workbooks?

Often people use these workbooks because they want to find out more about why they feel as they do, and to find out how to make changes.

As part of feeling anxious, people often have a sense of not being in control. In this course, **you, the reader, are in control** – and you can work on things at a time that suits you. Time and time again, people are surprised to see the amount of change they can make themselves using workbooks like this.

These workbooks use an approach called cognitive behavioural therapy (also called CBT, a kind of talking treatment). Don't worry though – there won't be any more jargon like that in the rest of the course. But you need to know that the course uses the CBT approach.

Lots of research has shown that self-help materials based on the CBT approach work well for problems such as anxiety, stress and panic attacks (these terms are all described in more detail later in this workbook). Also, CBT self-help is recommended for use in the National Health Service (NHS) in the UK as a treatment for these problems. A large research study on a companion book in this series has shown that the approach works very well as a treatment. People using the book felt better and were more able to live their wlives as they wanted to.

In this course, each workbook will teach you how to make changes in different areas of your life in clear, step-by-step ways.

Getting going

Well done! You have done something that quite a few people struggle to do – **you are still reading**.

Starting to change can sometimes seem a really hard thing to do. Have you ever bought or been given a book or a DVD and never even opened it or taken the wrapper off? Using this course is no different. In fact, in some ways it's harder because it's not a book that's there for entertainment. Instead these are **work**books – which aim to help you to change how you feel.

What should you read first?

People usually start the course by working through these two workbooks:

- This one – *Tackling your anxiety: starting out (... and how to keep going if you feel stuck).*
- And another workbook from Part 1 of this book – either *Understanding worry and stress* or *Understanding panic and phobias.*

The two *Understanding* workbooks will help you to start working out how your anxiety is affecting important areas of your life. They will also help you decide which other course workbooks you might need to use.

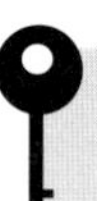

Key point

Remember **you** choose which workbooks you should work through – so make sure that you choose the ones that deal with the problems **you** are facing.

The different ways anxiety can affect you

Anxiety tends to affect people in the same sort of way again and again. For example, you may always get a headache or eyestrain when you become anxious. Others notice their anxiety in other ways:

- You may start to worry over even little problems and turn things over in your mind again and again.
- Or you may become very anxious and start to panic.

In the following few pages, you will find out more about the different ways that anxiety can affect you. After reading through these, you will be able to make a choice about which workbook to read next.

What are worry and stress?

Worrying thoughts are common in people with anxiety. When you are worried, you anxiously go over things again and again in a way that is unhelpful. Worrying is unhelpful because **it doesn't actually help you sort out the things that you are worried about**.

You may worry about things that have happened in the **past**, things happening **now**, or things that you think you might face in the **future**. Sometimes the worry may be out of all proportion. For example, you may worry for days or weeks over something that your partner or a friend said ages ago. So, even though whatever was said may have taken only a little bit of time, your worrying can add up to many days or even weeks. And with time, people often also find that they aren't too sure any more what exactly they are worrying about.

If you tend to worry about a lot of things in life, you feel stressed. This is called having *generalised anxiety*. Overall, about every one in 12 people feel stressed. This means that several people in your own road/street also probably have problems to do with stress at the same time as you.

The following checklist will help you recognise whether you have any of the common symptoms of stress.

Worry and stress checklist

Q Am I worried about things on most days?

Yes ☐ No ☐ Sometimes ☐

Q Do I find it hard to stop worrying?

Yes ☐ No ☐ Sometimes ☐

Q Am I anxiously going over things again and again in my mind in a way that hasn't actually helped me sort out my problems?

Yes ☐ No ☐ Sometimes ☐

Q Have I become too sensitive to possible problems

Yes ☐ No ☐ Sometimes ☐

Q Am I downplaying my own ability to overcome these problems?

Yes ☐ No ☐ Sometimes ☐

Q Do anxious worries make me tense and feel on edge?

Yes ☐ No ☐ Sometimes ☐

Q Do I feel mentally and physically tired as a result of my worry?

Yes ☐ No ☐ Sometimes ☐

Q Do I have problems sleeping because of worry?

Yes ☐ No ☐ Sometimes ☐

Q Have anxious thoughts caused me to reduce or stop what I do?

Yes ☐ No ☐ Sometimes ☐

Q Have worrying thoughts caused me to avoid dealing with my problems or people?

Yes ☐ No ☐ Sometimes ☐

If you have answered 'Yes' or 'Sometimes' to several of these questions, worry and stress are problems for you.

Key point

Next step: Try not to give up now and finish reading this workbook. If you do this, you can then start reading the *Understanding worry and stress* workbook to help you start getting rid of these problems.

What are panic attacks?

Sometimes your anxiety can rise to such a high level that you might feel mentally and physically tense and unwell. You may stop what you are doing and try to leave or escape the situation.

People sometimes even feel paralysed into inactivity. Think about how rabbits caught in the headlamps of a car just freeze, expecting disaster to strike at any moment. This sudden feeling of a lot of fear, dread or terror is called a *panic attack*. Panic attacks usually last about 20–40 minutes.

When people panic, they strongly believe that something terrible or catastrophic is happening **right now**. Common fears that people feel in a panic attack are:

- 'I'm going to faint.'
- 'I'm going to suffocate.'
- 'I'm going to collapse.'
- 'I'm going to have a stroke.'
- 'I'm going to have a heart attack.'

Sometimes the fear is of *going mad* or *losing control*. People feel immediately threatened or very scared and quickly stop what they are doing. They try to quickly get away from the situation.

Occasionally you may not feel fear or anxiety about anything in particular, but you can still get a panic attack. This usually happens when some other upsets or fears build up in your mind. At least one in 10 people have a panic attack at some time in their life.

Here's a checklist for you to try to recognise if you get panic attacks.

Panic attack checklist

Q Do I notice anxiety that rises to a peak?

Yes ☐ No ☐ Sometimes ☐

Q Do I feel very scared and physically unwell during the panic attack?

Yes ☐ No ☐ Sometimes ☐

Q Do I fear that something terrible or catastrophic will happen during that time?

Yes ☐ No ☐ Sometimes ☐

Q Do I become convinced that things that I fear might happen during the panic attack?

Yes ☐ No ☐ Sometimes ☐

Q Do I stop what I am doing and try to immediately escape or leave when I feel like this?

Yes ☐ No ☐ Sometimes ☐

Q Am I downplaying my own ability to overcome these problems?

Yes ☐ No ☐ Sometimes ☐

If you have answered 'Yes' or 'Sometimes' to several of these questions, then panic may be a problem for you. Talk to your healthcare practitioner about this, if you haven't done before.

Key point

Next step: Try not to give up now and finish reading this workbook. If you do this, you can then start reading the *Understanding panic and phobias* workbook to help you start getting rid of these problems.

What is a phobia?

You may have a friend or relative who is very scared of creatures such as spiders, or of situations such as heights. You yourself may have such fears.

Sometimes people become so fearful that even just thinking about the situation that scares them can result in strong feelings of panic. You may avoid anything to do with that situation as a result. This means that your life may become increasingly restricted. People also often lose their confidence and become distressed for a very long time. When this occurs, it's described as having a **phobia**.

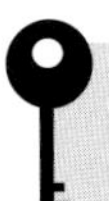

Key point

A *phobia* means having high levels of anxiety (often with panic attacks) regularly in a particular situation. You become overly aware of any possible threats linked to your fear. So you try to **avoid or quickly leave** any situation, people or places that cause you to feel anxious. Even though you may already know logically that the situation will not harm or kill you, you feel the anxiety anyway.

Virtually any situation, or people, or a place can cause phobia. The list below describes the main types of phobia.

- Avoiding particular **situations** or objects: A common example of situations that people avoid is a fear of heights. Almost any object can become a cause of phobic fear, for example insects, wasps, dogs, flies or spiders.
- Avoiding conversations with **people** or being in situations where you might think your performance is being judged, such as dancing. People who feel very shy or very high anxiety in social situations have what is called a **social phobia**. Sometimes the fear is to do with a particular thing, such as speaking to a large group of people. For example, a teacher may become anxious while talking to a class.
- Avoiding specific **places**. You may have heard of people who have panic attacks on buses or in shops or other crowded situations from where it is hard to escape quickly. This is called **agoraphobia**. It's one of the most common types of phobia.

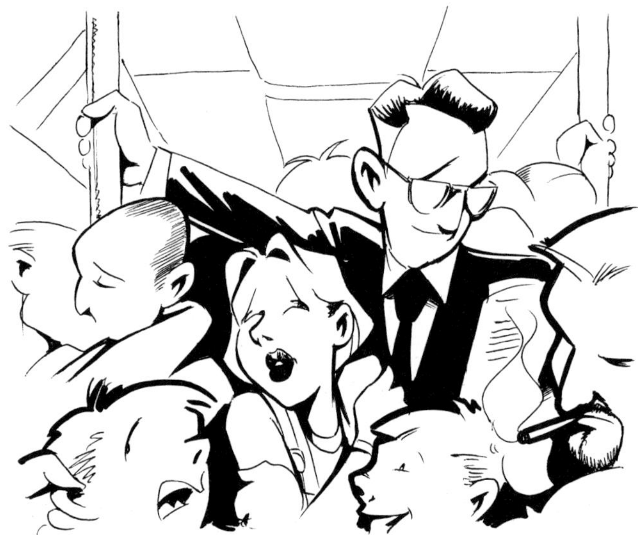

Phobias, worry, depression and panic attacks commonly happen together.

Here is a checklist to help you recognise if you may have a phobia.

Phobia checklist

Q Do I feel very anxious or do I panic when I face particular situations, people or places?

Yes ☐ No ☐ Sometimes ☐

Q Does even thinking about these situations, places or people make me feel nervous?

Yes ☐ No ☐ Sometimes ☐

Q Have I become too sensitive to anything to do with the phobic fear?

Yes ☐ No ☐ Sometimes ☐

Q Am I avoiding these situations, places or people so that I don't feel anxious?

Yes ☐ No ☐ Sometimes ☐

Q Overall, is my life becoming increasingly restricted as a result?

Yes ☐ No ☐ Sometimes ☐

Q Am I downplaying my own ability to overcome these fears?

Yes ☐ No ☐ Sometimes ☐

If you have answered 'Yes' or 'Sometimes' to any of these questions, then you may have a phobia. Talk to your healthcare practitioner about this.

Key point

Next step: Try not to give up now and finish reading this workbook. If you do this, you can then start reading the *Understanding panic and phobias* workbook to help you start getting rid of these problems.

Developing a routine in using the workbooks

Have you ever noticed how your surroundings can affect how you feel? For example, if you are used to having a snack while you watch television, sometimes just sitting in the same chair can make you feel hungry.

In the same way, you might find it helps to set aside a particular place to complete the workbooks. For example, sitting on a chair at the kitchen table (your 'workbook chair') with a pen and some blank paper to jot down ideas as you read. It also makes sense to try to plan enough time to read – preferably half an hour or so at a time. This will help you concentrate better on the workbook. If you have others around you, like young children who might interrupt, try to choose a time when they are asleep or away at nursery or school. Or perhaps a friend or a relative could help look after them for the time you are working on the course?

Planning how and when to use the workbooks

It is often helpful to actively plan doing the course into your day or your diary rather than just 'trying to fit it in sometime'. The best plans say:

- What you are going to do.
- When you are going to do it.

and

- **Predict** things that might block or get in the way of you doing this.

You may find the following **Planning task** helpful in making this regular commitment. You can use it to help you plan how to use the next workbook.

Your plan to use the workbooks

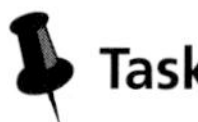

Task

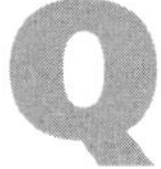

When are you going to read the next workbook?

Is reading some of the workbook every day practical for you? If not every day, is every other day more realistic? Write the day and time when you plan to do this here:

Do you feel more able to concentrate at a particular time of day? For example, many people with low mood notice they feel at their worst first thing in the morning. You might therefore find that the best time for you to read the workbooks is after lunch, in the late afternoon, or in the early evening. If you have young children, think about their routine. Or you could pick a time when others are around to help look after them.

How much will you read at a time?

You may find it easier to read just a few pages at a time – making sure that you stop, think and reflect by answering the questions as you do this. Each workbook is also split up into sections that you can work through in chunks one at a time to help this process.

Write down your plan of how much you will read here:

Is your plan realistic, practical and achievable?

You know your own life and its various demands and commitments, so this is a question only you can answer.

What problems could block or prevent you doing this course, and how can you overcome those problems?

Unexpected things may happen from time to time, and interrupt your plans. Have a back-up time planned for if you can't start working on the course when you first planned. For example, what if a friend drops by for a coffee, or (if you have one) your baby cries, wakes up or needs a nappy change. Write your possible blocks in here:

How can you unblock them?

Getting into the mood: doing something physical can help you get started

You may feel physically and mentally sluggish when you are stressed or when you aren't sleeping well. You might be doing very little during the day, and it may be hard to see yourself making any changes.

A good start to using the workbooks is to do something physical first. For example, get up and walk around the room or up and down the stairs, if you have them. Then sit down on your 'workbook chair' – such as a kitchen chair that forces you to sit upright rather than slump back. Now start reading the workbook. Have some pens and paper with you so you can make notes and write in the workbook.

Writing in the workbook

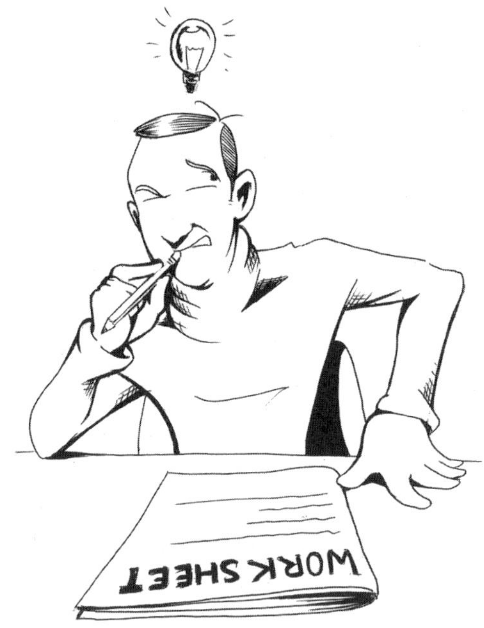

Things can look different when you write them down. You can notice patterns and habits you might otherwise have missed. Therefore, try to answer all the questions as you go through the different workbooks. Answer them straight away rather than thinking you will come back to it later.

You might not wish to write in the book – it may be something you don't like to do or you may have borrowed the book from a library or someone else. If so, you can write your answers on a separate sheet of paper. Many of the blank sheets in the book are available to print off free of charge from **www.fiveareas.com**.

But my life is too busy/unpredictable to use the course

All this sounds very straightforward, doesn't it? But sometimes life can be busy or unpredictable. To begin with, your first step might well be a case of taking the time when you can. Or perhaps sometimes someone else can come round and help out while you work on things.

Here are some suggestions of how to build on this first step during the rest of the course.

Some dos and don'ts for getting the most out of the course

Do:

- Try to work through one workbook a week.
- Get a pen. Writing things down means you are thinking and learning. In fact it's more than that. Sometimes you actually work out what you really think about something when you write it down.
- Answer all the questions – and do try to stop, think and reflect as you read.
- Ask: How does this apply to me? How might I use this in my life?
- Try out what you read in the workbooks. It can be tempting when we feel anxious to put things off, but putting things off will mean nothing changes. There is a section at the end of each workbook that will help you to decide how to do this. Have you any ideas so far? Take what helps and use it again and again.
- Be realistic. You are more likely to succeed if you try changing things one step at a time rather than throwing yourself into things and then running out of steam. Having realistic goals is another way of making sure you don't end up feeling too scared to make any changes at all.
- Make notes in the 'My notes' section at the end of each workbook or on a sheet of paper. Also re-read sections of the workbooks and your notes to go over what you have learned. You may find that different parts become clearer, or seem more useful on reading a second time.
- Use the workbooks to build on the help you receive in other ways, such as talking to friends, or from self-help organisations and support groups.
- Say 'well done' to yourself and tell others you are making progress.

Don't:

- Expect a sudden miracle cure. Change takes time and practice.
- Try to do this completely on your own. Supportive encouragement from a trusted friend, health professional or social care worker can really help.
- Try to read the workbook against the odds, such as the times when you are trying to do other tasks.
- Cut yourself off from other useful supports. You can do this course alongside other treatments, such as seeing your doctor or other health or social care workers. These approaches can all be helpful parts of moving forwards.

Finding extra support

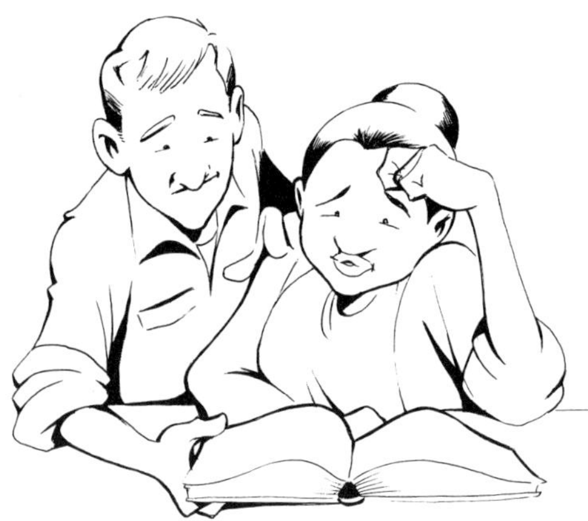

Having someone around who can offer *support and encouragement* can help. This is especially important if you feel you are struggling or feel stuck. Sometimes just the act of telling someone – a family member, friend or health worker – that you are working on something, or plan to do a certain activity on a particular day can really help. Just knowing that someone else may ask you how it's going could help spur you into action. You might go through your answers to the questions in the workbooks with them – or keep your answers private and only discuss some of the course content.

Many people find it helpful to have a healthcare practitioner to support them and keep a check on how things are going. This can be done either face to face or even by talking on the telephone or by email. If you can do this, it is a very good way of working with the CBT approach. Otherwise, ask your own doctor if he or she would be willing to support you about two or three times over the next month or so just for a short review of your progress to encourage you to use this approach.

Building your motivation to change

At times of anxiety, stress or a panic attack you may not feel motivated to do anything. You may be sleeping poorly, have low energy levels and struggle to be motivated to change.

It might help if you write yourself the following **letter**. Try to do this now, before moving on, even if it seems hard to do.

Imagine it is 10 years in the future. You have made important changes in your life and things are much better. Write yourself an **encouraging letter** about why you need to make changes now. Keeping the letter and reread it wherever you feel you need extra encouragement.

Dear (your name)

Signed:

(Myself)

Change takes time

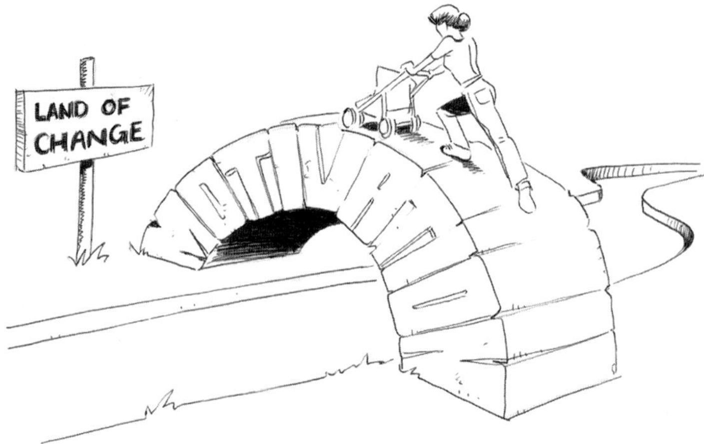

Sometimes it's easy to forget how hard it is to learn new information or skills that you now take for granted. Think about some of the skills you have learned over the years. For example, if you can drive or swim or ride a bike, think back to your first driving/swimming lesson or attempt to cycle without stabilisers. You probably weren't very good at it that first time, yet with practice you developed the skills needed to do it. In the same way, you can help improve how you feel by practising what you learn – even if it may seem hard at first.

Write down some other things you have learnt that took time

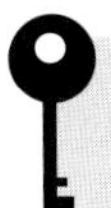

Key point

You can't expect to be able to swim immediately. You may need to start at the shallow end and practise at first. Use the workbooks in a similar way. Pace what you do and don't jump straight away into the deep end.

Having realistic expectations

It's important not to approach this course either far too positively or far too negatively. It would be untrue to claim that if you use this course you are guaranteed results. What we can guarantee is that this Five Areas Approach has helped many thousands of people – and that the workbooks teach clinically proved approaches that have been a help for many. Hopefully, at the very least you will learn some interesting and helpful things along the way.

Common problems in using the course

I've no time

Life can be busy and complicated – especially if you have family or work commitments. There will be many demands on your time. But ...

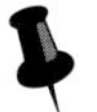

Task

Imagine you have a close friend who is troubled by anxious fears. They don't like how they feel – and you know that it's affecting them in lots of different ways. What helpful advice would you give them if they said 'I've no time'.

Write down your encouraging advice here:

... if you would give your friend this advice to make some time – could you use that same advice yourself?

I feel too stressed to do this now

Sometimes if we feel particularly bad it might not be the right time to use these workbooks. But you can always come back to them later if you are finding that things are too much now. If you can't concentrate for long because of feeling anxious or stressed, just go at a pace you can manage. You should also discuss any other treatment options with your doctor or other healthcare or social worker.

I'll never change

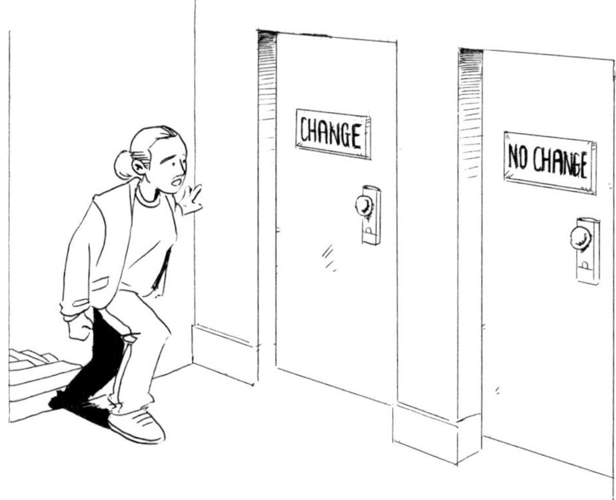

One big block to getting better is not believing that you can change. Many people find that they gain much more from the course than they first thought they would. Could this be true for you?

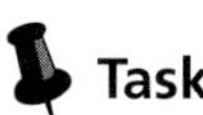 **Task**

Again, imagine if your friend told you they believed they would never change from a time of distress. They need encouragement.

What words of encouragement would you say to your friend? Write them down here:

If you would offer helpful and positive advice to a friend, then why not also offer it to yourself?

Experiment

Even if you have doubts about the course, or about your ability to use it effectively, try to give it a go. In this way you can test it out in your own life. If you still find it doesn't help after you've given it a good go, it would be a sensible time to try something different.

Summary

Well done – you've got to the last section – and you're still reading! That's a very important achievement. So many people who want to change find it hard starting out.

Let's review what you have learned in this workbook. You have covered:

- How to get the most out of the course.
- How to write a clear but flexible plan of when to use the workbooks.
- How to overcome common blocks to change.

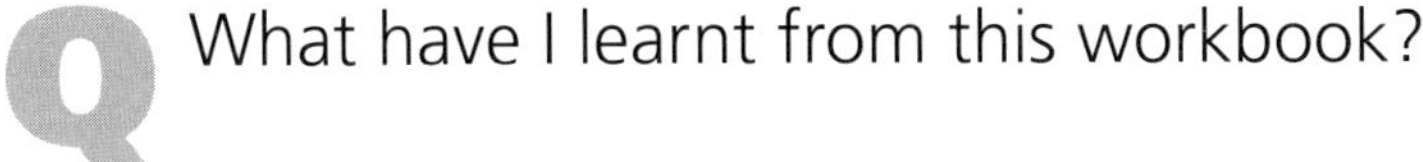

What have I learnt from this workbook?

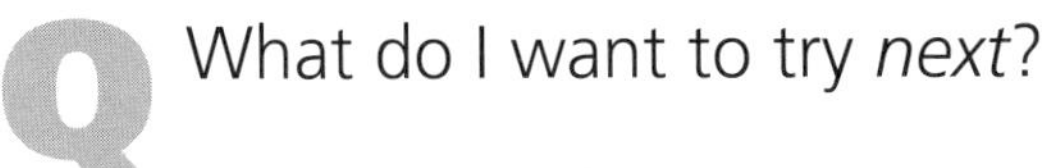

What do I want to try *next*?

Putting into practice what you have learned

You are likely to make the most progress if you can put into practice what you have learned in the workbook. Each workbook will encourage you to do this by suggesting certain tasks for you to do in the following days.

Suggested practice plan

Read one of the two *Understanding* workbooks next. Use the **Planning task** on page 51 to plan this. These workbooks will help you work out which other course workbooks are relevant to you.

Other sources of support

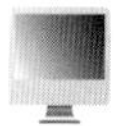

www.livinglifetothefull.com

This popular website is designed to support readers of this workbook and is free to use. You will need to register and then log in every time you wish to use it. The website teaches people how to use the various resources written by Dr Chris Williams, and is supported by various organisations including charities and the NHS in Scotland. But it's free to access by anyone, wherever they live. Many other resources for support are also available for people who get anxious, stressed or have panic attacks. These are listed on the Living Life to the Full website.

www.fiveareas.com

This second website also provides access to other Five Areas books and resources, including free handouts and resources such as relaxation MP3 files. Translations of the resources in various languages and large print versions that can be read by screen readers are available via the website.

A request for feedback

An important part in the development of all the Five Areas Approach workbooks is that the content is updated on a regular basis based on feedback from users and practitioners. If there are areas in this course that you find hard to understand, or seemed poorly written, please let us know (see contact details below). However, we can't answer specific questions or provide advice on treatment.

Address: Five Areas, PO Box 9, Glasgow G63 0WL, UK.

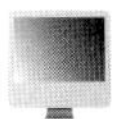

Our website: **www.fiveareas.com**
email: **feedback@fiveareas.com**

Acknowledgements

The cartoon illustrations in the workbooks have been produced by Keith Chan (kchan75@hotmail.com).

My notes

Overcoming Anxiety, Stress and Panic

A Five Areas Approach

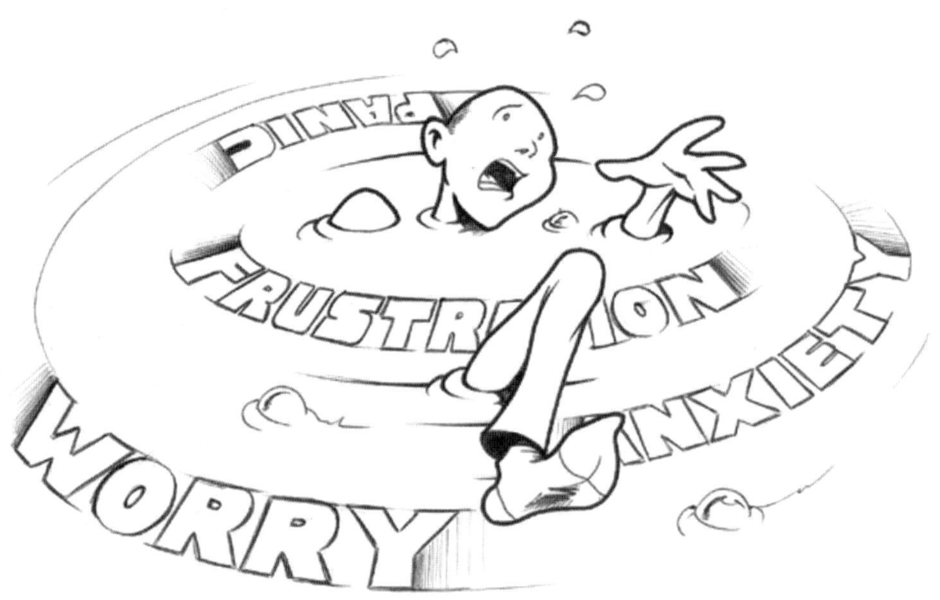

Understanding worry and stress

www.livinglifetothefull.com
www.fiveareas.com

Dr Chris Williams

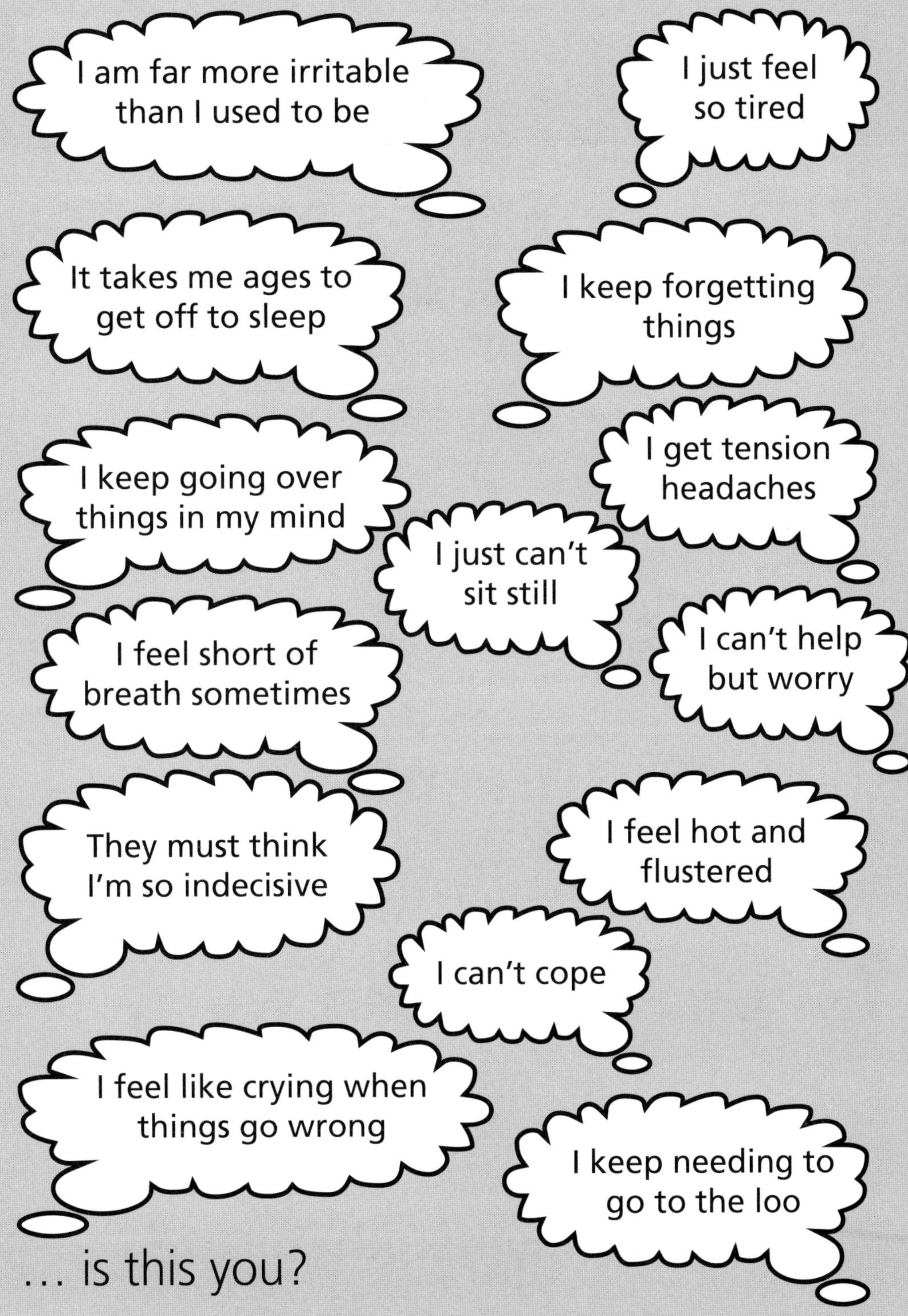
I am far more irritable than I used to be
I just feel so tired
It takes me ages to get off to sleep
I keep forgetting things
I keep going over things in my mind
I get tension headaches
I just can't sit still
I feel short of breath sometimes
I can't help but worry
They must think I'm so indecisive
I feel hot and flustered
I can't cope
I feel like crying when things go wrong
I keep needing to go to the loo

… is this you?

If it is … this **workbook is for you**.

This workbook will help you to:

- Understand what anxiety, worry and stress are.
- Recognise how these conditions can affect you.
- Identify the areas you need to tackle to overcome your own problems of anxiety.

Understanding anxiety

The words *stressed*, *hassled*, *tense* and *worry* all describe a situation of anxiety. Anxiety is a normal and common feeling (emotion) that can be helpful even though it can feel unpleasant. For example, a small amount of anxiety can help motivate some people to prepare for events such as interviews and exams, and even in crossing the road. Anxiety is also helpful in situations of sudden danger, where it helps you to respond and get away as quickly as possible.

Anxiety becomes a problem when people feel:

- Anxious in situations that are not dangerous at all.
- Extremely anxious – well beyond what is helpful anxiety. For example, being so worried about things that you can't get off to sleep.

What are worry and stress?

Worrying thoughts are common in anxiety.

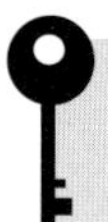

Key point

When people worry, they anxiously go over things again and again in a way that is unhelpful. This is because it doesn't actually help sort out the problems that they are worried about.

Worry causes you to think again and again about things that happened in the past. You may also worry about things in the present or what might happen in the future. This type of constant, anxious worrying is sometimes called stress. It's also sometimes described as having *generalised anxiety*, that is, people feel generally anxious about very many things in life.

Often, people don't want to talk about mental health problems. So you may think you are the only person to have these problems. But this isn't true. You may be surprised to learn that there are possibly at least one or two people living near to you, in your street, who also have problems with anxiety. The following checklist will help you to recognise whether you have any of the common symptoms of anxious worrying. As you are reading this workbook, you will probably have already gone through the checklist in the *Tackling your anxiety: starting out (... and how to keep going if you feel stuck)* workbook. If you had answered 'Yes' or 'Sometimes' to several of the questions in that checklist, then anxiety is a problem for you.

Worry and stress checklist

Q Am I worried about things on most days?

Yes ☐ No ☐ Sometimes ☐

Q Do I find it hard to stop worrying?

Yes ☐ No ☐ Sometimes ☐

Q Am I anxiously going over things again and again in my mind in a way that doesn't help me sort out my problems?

Yes ☐ No ☐ Sometimes ☐

Q Have I become too sensitive to possible problems?

Yes ☐ No ☐ Sometimes ☐

Q Do anxious worries make me tense and feel on edge?

Yes ☐ No ☐ Sometimes ☐

Q Do I feel mentally and physically tired as a result of my worry?

Yes ☐ No ☐ Sometimes ☐

Q Do I have problems sleeping because of worry?

Yes ☐ No ☐ Sometimes ☐

Q Have anxious thoughts caused me to reduce or stop what I do?

Yes ☐ No ☐ Sometimes ☐

Q Have worrying thoughts caused me to avoid dealing with my problems or people?

Yes ☐ No ☐ Sometimes ☐

Q Am I downplaying my own ability to cope?

Yes ☐ No ☐ Sometimes ☐

If you have answered 'Yes' or 'Sometimes' to several of these questions, anxiety is a problem for you.

Worrying thoughts can also occur alongside other problems such as:

- *Panic attacks* – people may have panic attacks when they are extremely anxious or full of fear. If you think this could happen to you, the workbook *Understanding panic and phobias* will help you find out more about these conditions.
- *Depression* – people who are depressed often also tend to have anxious worrying. The depressing thoughts are linked in with low mood, a lack of enjoyment and reduced activity. If you think you may be depressed, you should talk to your healthcare practitioner to find out more about being depressed.

The first step of working out how to make changes is to see how things have developed over time. Understanding how things have changed can help you get a clearer idea of how anxiety and stress are affecting you now. It can also help you work out what aspects of life you want to work on so as to get back to feeling better again.

How did things get to be like this?

Anyone can feel stressed if their emotional balance is upset. You can use a time line to find out how you started to feel this way. An example is shown below.

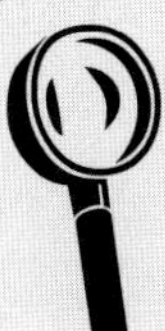

Example: Helen's time line

Helen works from home as a book-keeper and lives with her partner Paul.

- Beginning:

  January: Paul started to have problems with depression. He needed more support.

  February: Paul was struggling, and I started to find it hard to care for him and do my job as a book-keeper. I began to feel stressed and tense and was sleeping badly.

  April: Paul was struggling at work, and our relationship was struggling too. We were both increasingly ratty with each other. I was worried not only about him but also whether he would keep his job.

  June: Paul went off work sick. I was feeling stretched having to take on more work to keep our income up. Also, we were arguing more and now he's at home all day we are on top of each other which is making things worse.

  August: I felt I wasn't coping, near tears at times, happy at others. Not sleeping and not as hungry as before. My GP is suggesting that I should see a mental health practitioner. I feel so stressed.

- Today:

  I have started using the course workbooks – I want to make some changes.

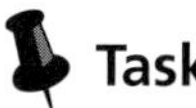

Task

Now it's your turn. Fill in your own time line below.

Beginning (a time when I didn't feel too worried, anxious or stressed):

Today:

The good news is that your time line doesn't stop here. If you can make changes, you will move forwards and bring back the balance in your life.

So the next step then is to see how worry and stress are affecting you.

Feeling out of balance – when worry or stress starts to get worse and worse

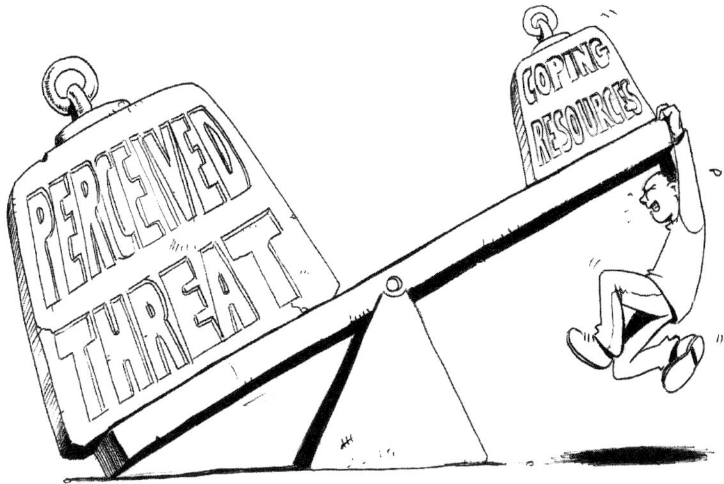

Normally, most people feel **able to cope** with the problems they face. When you are in balance, you know you can deal with your problems. So it isn't your situation or problem alone that causes you to feel worried or stressed. Instead it's how you think about these things that makes you feel like you do. And dwelling on problems and getting things out of perspective doesn't help you feel better or make your problem go away.

Q Do I feel in balance at the moment?

Yes ☐ No ☐ Sometimes ☐

If you feel out of balance some or all of the time, this course can help you get your balance back.

Let's start by finding out more about the Five Areas Approach. This can help you understand how worry and stress are affecting your life.

Understanding how you feel using the Five Areas Approach

One helpful way of understanding how worry or stress affects you is to think of the ways that it affects the different areas of your life. The **Five Areas Approach** can help you to do this by looking in detail at five important areas of your life.

The Five Areas are:

- **Area 1: People and events around you**. This includes the situations you face and people or places you find particularly hard to cope with.
- **Area 2: Your thinking**. This can often become extreme and unhelpful when you feel too worried or stressed. In worry, people over-estimate how hard things are, and under-estimate their ability to cope with things. They also dwell on things. They try to persuade themselves that thinking too much helps them sort out their problems. But turning worries over again and again and again doesn't help sort anything out.
- **Area 3: Your feelings (also called moods or emotions)**. You can feel tense, anxious, irritable, low, ashamed or guilty when you are stressed.
- **Area 4: Any altered physical symptoms in your body**. For example, you may feel shaky, sweaty or restless or you may notice tenseness or tightness in your body. These are described in more detail later.
- **Area 5: Your altered behaviour or activity levels**. This includes both – the helpful things you can do to make you feel better, and the unhelpful things you do, which backfire and make you feel even worse.

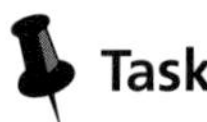

Task

Try to think about how the Five Areas assessment can help Helen understand how she is feeling.

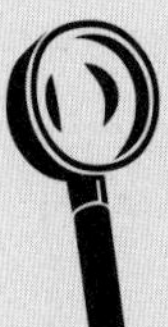

Example: How worry and stress are affecting Helen's life

The figure below shows how Helen's problems can be summarised using the Five Areas Approach.

Helen's Five Areas assessment

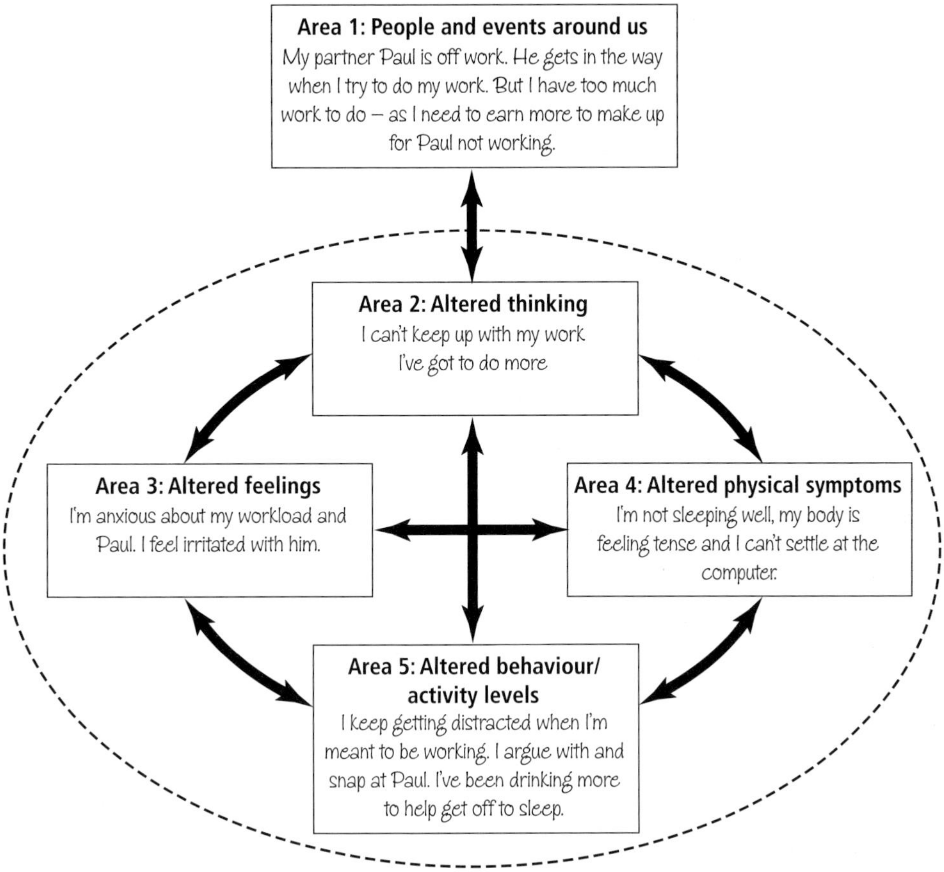

Area 1: People and events around us
My partner Paul is off work. He gets in the way when I try to do my work. But I have too much work to do – as I need to earn more to make up for Paul not working.

Area 2: Altered thinking
I can't keep up with my work
I've got to do more

Area 3: Altered feelings
I'm anxious about my workload and Paul. I feel irritated with him.

Area 4: Altered physical symptoms
I'm not sleeping well, my body is feeling tense and I can't settle at the computer.

Area 5: Altered behaviour/ activity levels
I keep getting distracted when I'm meant to be working. I argue with and snap at Paul. I've been drinking more to help get off to sleep.

The Five Areas diagram shows that what you think about a situation or problem can affect how you feel physically and emotionally. It also shows that your thinking affects what you do (your behaviour or activity levels). Look at the arrows in the diagram. All of the Five Areas of your life affect each other.

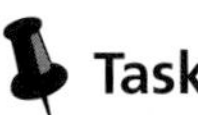

Task

Let's take a look at what's happening for you in each of the Five Areas, starting with Area 1.

Area 1: People and events around you

All of us from time to time face practical problems such as:

- Problems with family and life at home.
- The challenges of bringing up young children.

- Problems in relationships with partners or friends or colleagues.
- Other life challenges, for example problems at work, college, etc.

People who have had a relationship split, or who have no one to talk to, can feel very anxious, worried or stressed. Mothers facing the demands of trying to bring up young children are also at greater risk of anxiety, worry and stress.

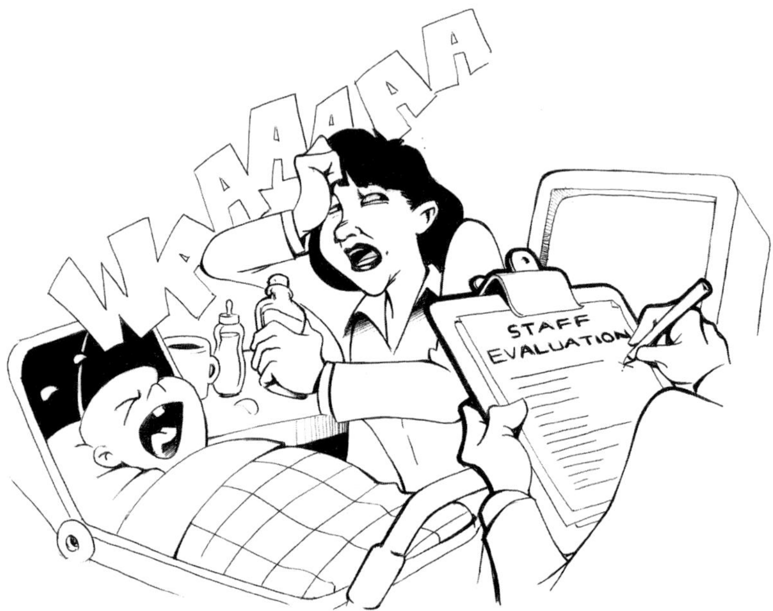

Worry, stress and anxiety can affect any kind of relationship. You may become confused about your feelings towards others, and you can lose interest in your relationships. Love can feel subdued. Similarly, those with a spiritual faith may feel they struggle to get the support that they usually get from their faith.

Are any of these relevant to you?

- There is no-one around who I can really talk to.

  Yes ☐ No ☐ Sometimes ☐

- I am struggling to cope with my work.

  Yes ☐ No ☐ Sometimes ☐

- My baby isn't feeding/sleeping easily.

  Yes ☐ No ☐ Sometimes ☐

- I worry about work or money or debts.

  Yes ☐ No ☐ Sometimes ☐

- There are problems where I live.

  Yes ☐ No ☐ Sometimes ☐

- My children won't do what I tell them.

  Yes ☐ No ☐ Sometimes ☐

- It's hard to get on with another person or people in my family.

  Yes ☐ No ☐ Sometimes ☐

- I am having problems with my neighbours.

  Yes ☐ No ☐ Sometimes ☐

- I have problems with colleagues at work.

  Yes ☐ No ☐ Sometimes ☐

- I/My family has unemployment worries.

  Yes ☐ No ☐ Sometimes ☐

- I/My family has housing problems.

  Yes ☐ No ☐ Sometimes ☐

Task

Now make a list of any other problems you may have. You may also find it helpful to write in some more detail about any of the problems you noted in the list above. Use an extra sheet of paper if you need to, or use the **My Notes** section at the end of this workbook.

Summary for Area 1: People and events around you

Now rate the extent of your problems in this area.

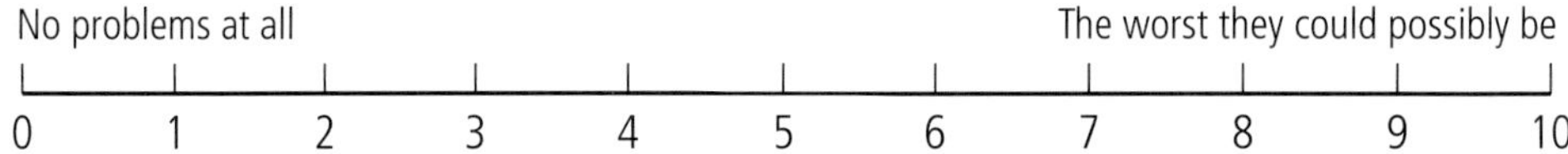

What next?

Looking at your score, check whether the people and events around you (your situation) is an area you wish to work on. If you do, two of the workbooks in the course will help you to tackle difficulties in this area:

- *How to ask for what you really need (being assertive)* – this workbook deals with how to be assertive and rebalance relationships.
- *How to start fixing problems and finding solutions (practical problem solving).*

Area 2: Your thinking

When someone feels very anxious, worried or stressed, how they **think** tends to change. You tend to lose confidence and find it harder to make decisions. You may worry about things you have done – and things you haven't done. You begin to see everything in quite negative or anxiety-provoking ways.

So your thinking becomes:

- Extreme.
- Unhelpful.

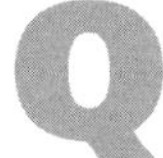

Have you noticed any of these common unhelpful patterns of thinking in your life?

Unhelpful thinking pattern	Do you ever think this way? (Put a tick in the box if you have noticed this thinking style – even if just sometimes.) Write down an example
Being your own worst critic/bias against yourself. For example, overlooking your strengths; seeing yourself as not coping; or not recognising your achievements	☐
Putting a negative slant on things (negative mental filter). For example, seeing things through dark-tinted glasses; seeing the glass as being half empty rather than half full; thinking that whatever you do in the week it's never enough to give you a sense of achievement; tending to focus on the bad side of everyday situations	☐
Have a gloomy view of the future. For example thinking that things will stay bad or get even worse; predicting that things will go wrong; or always looking for the next thing to fail	☐
Jumping to the worst conclusion. For example, predicting that the very worst outcome will happen, thinking that you will fail very badly	☐
Having a negative view about how others see you (mind-reading). For example, often thinking that others don't like you or think badly of you for no particular reason	☐
Unfairly taking responsibility for things. For example, thinking you should take the blame if things go wrong; feeling guilty about things that are not really your fault; and thinking that you are responsible for everyone else	☐
Making extreme statements/rules. For example using the words '*always*' or '*never*' a lot to summarise things; if a bad thing happens, saying '*just typical*' because it seems this always happens; making yourself a lot of '*must*', '*should*', '*ought*' or '*got to*' rules; believing you must always push yourself to do things well	☐

As explained before in this workbook, what you think can affect how you feel.

Example: How your thinking affects how you feel and what you do

People or events around us	Anxious thought	Unhelpful thinking style	Emotional and/or physical impact of the thinking	Behaviour change
The amount of work Helen needs to do is building up. She isn't going to meet the next deadline for her client	*I'll never get it done. I can't cope. I'll let the client down*	Gloomy view of the future. Helen is also being her own worst critic	*Emotional*: anxious and irritable. *Physical*: feels physically tense. Can't settle. Not sleeping well	Helen is working longer and longer hours. She is going to bed late because of her long hours. She is getting into arguments with her partner Paul. She is drinking more to feel less tense
Usha has just arrived at a party	*I won't have anything to say*	Making negative predictions	*Emotional*: anxious and scared. *Physical*: feels physically tense, and notices her heart speeding up	Usha makes an excuse and goes to the toilet. *Avoidance*: Usha tries to sit in a corner by herself and doesn't chat. She leaves early.
Steve has some work to do. He can't complete one part of the task in the time that he should have	*It's all gone wrong*	Putting a negative slant on things (negative mental filter)	*Emotional*: frustrated and annoyed at what he has to do, and at himself. *Physical*: feels tensed up and has shallow, rapid breathing whenever he thinks about the difficult task	Steve gives up trying to do the work. *Avoids* doing the same work again
Andrew is speaking to his manager. As he does so he worries what his manager really thinks of him	*Mr. Jones thinks I'm not working hard enough and wasting time*	*Mind reading*: second-guessing that others don't like him without actually checking if this is true	*Emotional*: anxious and tense. *Physical*: feels red, hot and sweaty	Andrew *unhelpfully* avoids eye contact as he talks. He brings the conversation to an abrupt end. He tries to *avoid* speaking to people, and starts to feel cut-off from everyone else (isolated)

In anxiety, people overplay the threat or danger that they are facing. And at the same time people usually downplay their capacity to cope with the problem. Little things that ordinarily wouldn't upset can really seem to strike home. Tears may be near to the surface.

You may think that you cannot cope with the demands you face, or the demands you place upon yourself. Things seem too much. There is no rest from the problems, nor can you stop thinking about them. Anxiety affects all aspects of your life. You may become clumsier and make more mistakes. Your attempts to get things right further add to anxiety and become just one more thing to beat yourself up about.

You may overlook your own strengths and be very self-critical. You may be prone to **mind read** and second-guess that others think negatively of you. But you may not check out whether these fears are true.

Overall, your thinking becomes extreme, unhelpful and out of all proportion. By thinking too much about problems that are taken out of all proportion, you tend to look down on your strengths and ability to cope. Things then seem as if they are out of control.

Images and mental pictures – an important part of anxiety

Sometimes people notice mental pictures or images in their mind when they become anxious. Images are a form of thought. They may be 'still' images (for example a photograph) or moving images (for example a video). Images may be in black and white or be in colour. They may include a mental picture of some worrying event occurring, such as someone reacting badly to a conversation you have had. As with all anxious fears, the images add to your feelings of anxiety.

Summary for Area 2: Your thinking

Rate the extent of your thinking problems here.

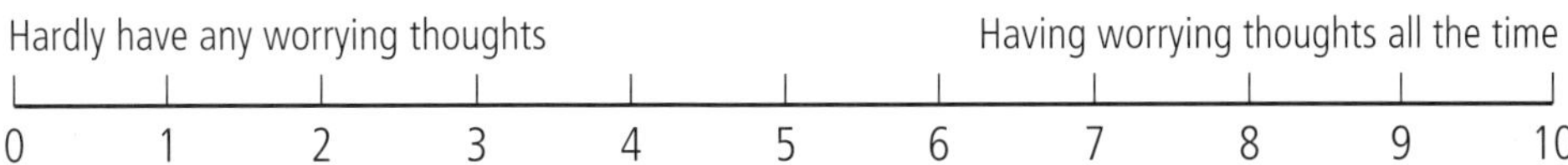

What next?

If this is an area you wish to work on, the *Noticing and changing anxious thinking* workbook will help you to find out and change these ways of thinking.

Area 3: Your feelings (emotions)

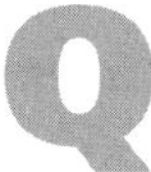

What emotional changes have you noticed over the past two weeks?

- Worry, stress or tension?

Yes ☐ No ☐ Sometimes ☐

- High levels of anxiety or panic (panic attacks)?

Yes ☐ No ☐ Sometimes ☐

- Lowness or sadness?

Yes ☐ No ☐ Sometimes ☐

- Reduced or no sense of pleasure in things?

Yes ☐ No ☐ Sometimes ☐

- Loss of all feelings, for example, noticing no feelings at all?

Yes ☐ No ☐ Sometimes ☐

- Guilt?

Yes ☐ No ☐ Sometimes ☐

- Anger or irritability (common if you are trying to escape during panic)?

Yes ☐ No ☐ Sometimes ☐

- Shame or embarrassment?

Yes ☐ No ☐ Sometimes ☐

- Other (write down here) changes in how you feel:

Your feelings (emotions) are an important and normal part of your life. Changes in how you feel are often linked with your thoughts, memories and the ideas that are going through your mind at the time. Try to become aware of these thoughts and note them down when there is a change in how you feel.

The good news is that by noticing these unhelpful changes you can begin to slowly make helpful changes in how you feel.

Summary for Area 3: Your feelings (emotions)

Rate the extent of how your feelings have changed on the graph below.

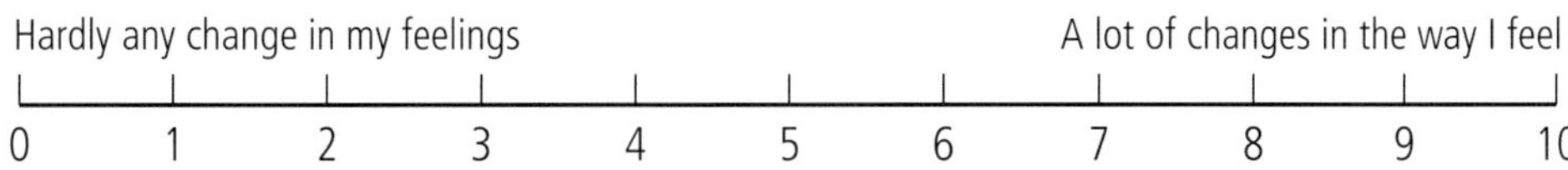

What next?

If this is an area you wish to work on, by making helpful changes in any of the other four areas you can change how you feel in a positive way.

Area 4: Altered physical symptoms

When a person becomes stressed, anxious or scared they notice a variety of physical changes.

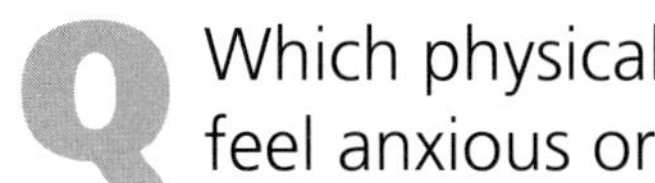

Which physical symptoms have you noticed when you feel anxious or stressed?

- Do you have a dry mouth?

Yes ☐ No ☐ Sometimes ☐

- Do you breathe too quickly with rapid, shallow breaths?

Yes ☐ No ☐ Sometimes ☐

- Do you notice a rapid or thumping heart?

Yes ☐ No ☐ Sometimes ☐

- Do you have a fuzzy-headed or faint feeling, or headaches?

Yes ☐ No ☐ Sometimes ☐

- Do your muscles get tense or do you feel restless or on edge (fidgety)?

  Yes ☐ No ☐ Sometimes ☐

- Do you feel shaky, hot or clammy and cold?

  Yes ☐ No ☐ Sometimes ☐

- Do you notice butterflies or a churning feeling in your stomach, or do you feel sick or get loose motions or go to the toilet frequently, or not feel hungry?

  Yes ☐ No ☐ Sometimes ☐

- Do you get pain, for example a painful chest, tummy or headaches – as if your head is in a vice or might explode?

  Yes ☐ No ☐ Sometimes ☐

- Do you notice a strong urge to wee or poo?

  Yes ☐ No ☐ Sometimes ☐

- Do you not feel like having sex or worry about your performance?

  Yes ☐ No ☐ Sometimes ☐

- Do you have any other symptoms?

Summary for Area 4: Altered physical symptoms

Having answered the questions, rate the extent of your problems in this graph.

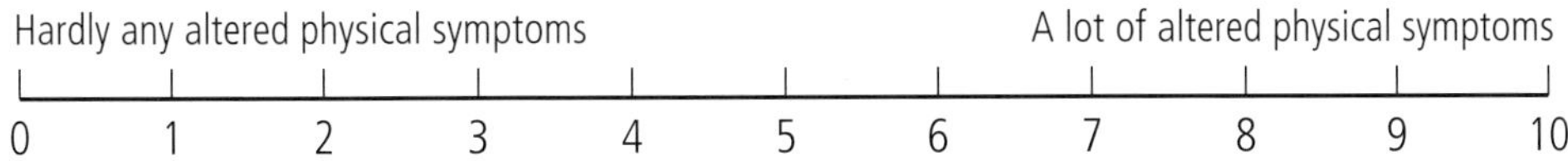

What next?

The good news is that by making changes in other areas, you can improve how you feel physically. You will find some helpful advice about how to tackle many of your physical symptoms in the *Overcoming anxious overbreathing (hyperventilation)* workbook. You can also download free relaxation recordings from **www.fiveareas.com**.

Area 5: Altered behaviour or activity levels

You have already worked hard in thinking about the first four of the five areas in your Five Areas assessment – well done! Here you look at the last area – altered behaviour (things that you can do).

Key point

Making changes in your behaviour and activity levels are some of the most helpful things you can do to boost how you feel and overcome anxiety.

Some things that you do can worsen how you feel. On the other hand, many ways in which you respond can be very helpful and boost how you are feeling. The ways in which your altered behaviours may worsen things are:

First type of altered behaviour: Reduced activity

When you feel stressed, tense or down, it's hard to keep doing things because you have:

- Low energy and feel tired ('I'm too tired').
- Little enjoyment or achievement when you do things.
- Negative thoughts about things ('I just can't be bothered').

All these lead to reduced activity – where you do less of or stop doing things **which are important** to you. Often the first things that are squeezed out are things that have previously given you a sense of **fun** or **achievement** (for example, meeting up with friends, and doing things with your family). You can also lose your sense of **closeness** to others.

It begins to seem as though everything is too much effort. And so you feel worse and worse.

Write down any examples of reduced activity you have noticed here:

The good news is that once you have noticed whether this is true for you, you can start working on your reduced activity in a planned, step-by-step way. You will find some suggestions for how to do this in the workbook *Facing fears and overcoming avoidance*.

Second type of altered behaviour: Avoiding or escaping from things

People often start to avoid or escape from people, places and situations that make them feel stressed. This may make you feel less anxious in the short term. But in the longer term, avoiding things makes it harder and harder to confidently face your fears in the future. And you don't see that your worst fears don't actually occur. In fact, avoidance teaches people the unhelpful rule that you only cope with a situation by avoiding it.

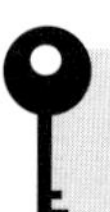

Key point

Avoidance and escaping can make you feel worse and also undermine your confidence.

Some things you may be avoiding

- Talking with people.
- Making decisions – or looking to others to make decisions for you.
- Saying that you disagree about something, or have a different opinion.
- Talking about how stressed and anxious you are feeling.
- Doing a task or going to a place that seems difficult and stressful.

Write down some examples of activities or things you have been avoiding:

The good news is that once you have noticed that you are tending to avoid things, you can start working on tackling avoidance and escaping. The workbook *Facing fears and overcoming avoidance* tells you how to do this.

Third type of altered behaviour: Dropping helpful things you do

Helpful behaviours include doing things such as:

- Talking to friends or family for support.
- Reading or using self-help materials or attending a self-help group.
- Going to see a doctor or healthcare practitioner.
- Finding activities or meeting people who give you a boost.
- If you have a personal spiritual faith, your beliefs may provide helpful support.

My helpful behaviours

Q Has anxiety, worry or stress caused you to stop doing activities that help you?

Yes ☐ No ☐ Sometimes ☐

Write down any examples of helpful behaviours you do (or have done before) here:

It is important to make time to keep doing these activities as they really do help.

Fourth type of altered behaviour: Unhelpful things you do

Sometimes people may do things that make them feel better at first but in the longer term, these things backfire and make you feel worse. Do you do any of the following unhelpful behaviours?

Trying to escape and hurry away:

- Rushing through a task so you can leave quickly.
- Walking more quickly than normal.
- Making an excuse, or lying and saying you are ill or have another urgent reason why you need to leave early or not attend.

Distracting yourself mentally by trying hard not to think about how you feel. For example:

- Trying desperately hard not to think about how you feel
- Trying to block how you feel by doing things that make you feel safer *mentally* (like doing maths sums or saying 'I'm all right' again and again or focusing on the lines on the floor) or through *actions* (such as biting your lip or digging your nails into your hand, gripping hard onto things for support).

Blocking anxiety using other approaches:

- Using alcohol or street drugs to block how you feel.
- Misusing prescribed medication by taking extra doses that are not prescribed to block how you feel.
- Asking someone to accompany you if you feel anxious.
- Seeking reassurance from others all the time.

Other unhelpful behaviours are:

- Withdrawing into yourself and cutting yourself off from your friends or family.
- Neglecting yourself (for example, by not eating as much or not washing).
- Finding yourself tempted to do things that you know are unwise or wrong. This might include deliberately taking risks, picking fights or betraying a partner.
- Harming yourself as a way of blocking how you feel (for example, self-cutting).
- Shouting or screaming at others out of frustration or getting angry if people seem to crowd or hassle you.

Write down any examples of unhelpful behaviour you do here:

The purpose of all the unhelpful behaviours is to feel safer/better – at least in the short term. Therefore, they are sometimes called *safety behaviours*. But, although safety behaviours may help you feel better in the short term, this doesn't last. **The anxiety returns to the same or even higher level**.

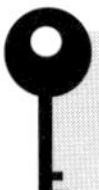

Key point

An important thing to watch out for is whether you have got into a habit of reacting to difficult situations in certain ways. By watching out for any unhelpful behaviours that you may have a tendency to fall into, and by choosing to respond differently, you can make large changes in how you are feeling.

You will find out more about reducing unhelpful behaviours in the workbook *Things you do that worsen your anxiety (unhelpful behaviours)*.

Summary for Area 5: Any altered behaviours/activity levels

Now think about all the altered behaviours you have identified and rate the extent of your problems in this area.

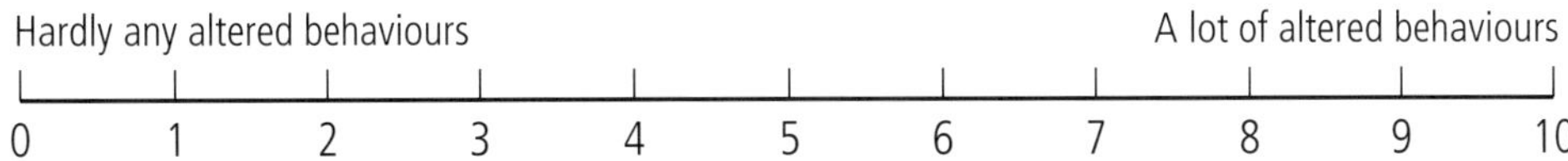

What next?

Remember that the purpose of the Five Areas Approach is to help you recognise how anxiety, worry or stress is affecting you. In this way, this approach can help you decide which areas you need to work on to bring about change.

The good news is that all the areas are linked so that making changes in any one area can lead to change in the others. So if you try to alter any one of these areas, it will help you tackle your problem.

Spotting patterns that affect your anxiety

The first thing is to do some research on how you are feeling.

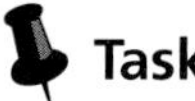

Use the Anxiety diary at the end of the workbook to record **all the times** when you feel too anxious, worried or stressed over the next week. You can download more pages for free from **www.fiveareas.com**. The aim is to play detective and recognise the things that are worsening the situation for you.

Then write down what you discover.

What seems to make you feel worse or better?

- Do certain situations seem to affect how bad your anxiety gets? (For example: going for an interview, being asked to do something at work, having too many things happening at once, or working to a deadline.)

- Do certain other feelings seem to affect how bad your anxiety gets? (For example, is it affected by feeling low, angry, guilty or ashamed?)

- Does thinking or worrying about particular fears make your anxiety worse?

- Does poor sleep or rapid breathing affect how you feel?

- Does doing exercise make your anxiety better?

- If you are using any medication, alcohol or street drugs, do you feel worse within a couple of hours of using them?

Identifying your early warning signs

Use your Anxiety diary to think back in detail about some of the recent times when you have felt more anxious or worried. Were there any early warning signs:

- Either that some things that bring on the anxiety were building up?
- Or that you were beginning to become anxious?

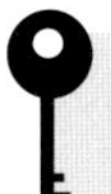

Key point

Early warning signs of anxiety include:

- Altered thinking: with anxious worries about things.
- Altered feelings: for example, with rising tension, dropping mood, becoming irritated or angry.
- Altered physical symptoms: for example, feeling fidgety, tossing and turning, feeling hot, sweaty or muscle tenseness.
- Altered behaviours or activity levels: for example, drinking more, walking faster, trying to leave a stressful situation, raising your voice, trying to avoid conversations.

By noticing your early warning signs you can choose to tackle the worrying thoughts before they start getting worse.

Where do you start?

The workbooks in this course can help you begin to tackle all of the five problem areas of anxiety and stress.

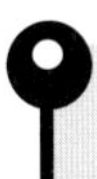

Key point

One key to success is to try **not to tackle everything at once**. You are more likely to improve by taking slow, steady steps. If you are too enthusiastic at the start and try to change too much together, you can run out of steam. So try to take things one step at a time by choosing and focusing on a particular area you are going to start with.

Set yourself:

- Short-term targets: these are changes you can make today, tomorrow and next week.
- Medium-term targets: these are changes to be put in place over the next few weeks.
- Long-term targets: this is where you want to be in six months or a year.

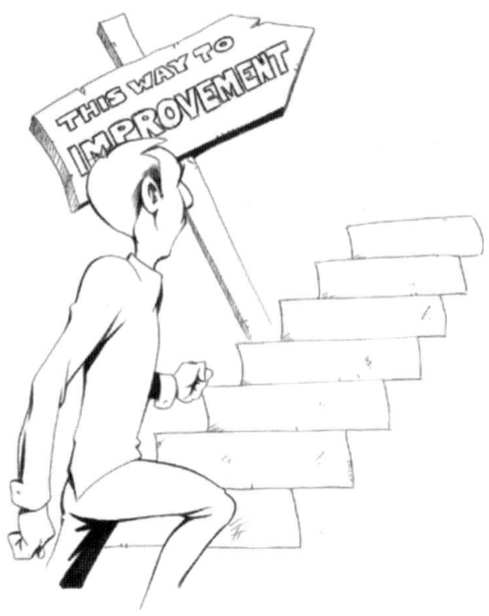

Which workbook should you try first?

Because each of the five areas of your life affects the other, choosing any of the areas to start on makes sense. Just choose something **you** want to work on now.

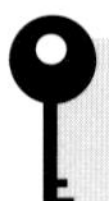

Key point

There isn't a set 'course' in this book. The course you take will include as many workbooks as you feel you need to use. Your Five Areas assessment will help you choose which workbook to read first.

In the table below, put a tick next to the workbooks you plan to read and also put a tick after you have completed it. Put a * by the first workbook you will work on.

Workbook	Plan to read	Tick when completed
Understanding why you feel as you do		
Tackling your anxiety: starting out (… and how to keep going if you feel stuck)	☐	☐
Understanding worry and stress	☐	☐
Understanding panic and phobias	☐	☐
Making changes to do with people and events around us		
How to start fixing problems and finding solutions (practical problem solving)	☐	☐
How to ask for what you really need (being assertive)	☐	☐
Learning to be calmer, less annoyed and less irritated	☐	☐
Making changes in your life		
How to get a good night's sleep: overcoming anxiety and sleep problems	☐	☐
Using exercise to overcome stress	☐	☐
Things you do that worsen your anxiety (unhelpful behaviours)	☐	☐
Stress, alcohol and drugs	☐	☐
Facing fears and overcoming avoidance	☐	☐
Understanding and overcoming shyness and social phobia	☐	☐
Noticing and changing anxious thinking	☐	☐
Understanding and overcoming feelings of depersonalisation	☐	☐
Overcoming anxious overbreathing (hyperventilation)	☐	☐

Two additional workbooks, *Understanding and using anti-anxiety medication* and *Planning for the future* are available free from **www.livinglifetothefull.com**.

Repeat your **Five Areas assessment** after using each workbook to help you decide where to go next.

How do I know if I need extra help?

Ideally, people using these workbooks will have someone to support them in doing it. But there are times when this won't be enough. If you struggle to do the tasks in the workbooks don't worry. Just do what you can. But if things *still* do not seem to be improving, you may need to get extra help.

If you have somebody supporting you, discuss what you have been doing with them. Otherwise make an appointment to see your doctor or a mental health worker.

Sources of extra help

You can ask:

- **Someone you can trust** – or you may find it easier to talk to someone *outside* your closest friends and family. Don't feel guilty if you want to do this – remember it's *normal* to feel like this.
- **Your family doctor or GP**.
- **Social services**. Social services can be a great source of support for families. You can find your local social services office hours' enquiry phone number and a 24-hour emergency phone number in the *Yellow Pages*.

Other organisations you can approach are:

- Anxiety UK: this charity has excellent online resources at **www.anxietyuk.org.uk**. There are forums and live chat as well as email support. The charity also has a helpline (**08444 775 774** – Monday to Friday 9.30am–5.30pm).
- Triumph over Phobia: this charity runs local groups for people with anxiety, panic and obsessive-compulsive problems. (See **www.topuk.org** or call **0845 600 9601** or email: info@topuk.org).
- Royal College of Psychiatrists: you can get fact sheets about anxiety and stress from the college's website (**www.rcpsych.ac.uk**) or by calling **020 7235 2351**.
- British Association for Behavioural and Cognitive Psychotherapies: the website of this organisation (**www.babcp.com**) has information about cognitive behaviour therapy and a list of accredited cognitive behaviour therapy practitioners and how to access them.

Other books that may be of help

You can get the following helpful books from local or online bookshops including **www.fiveareas.com** or you may find them at your local library:

- *Overcoming Depression and Low Mood: A Five Areas Approach*, third edition by C Williams.
- *Overcoming Teenage Depression and Low Mood: A Five Areas Approach* by N Dummett and C Williams.
- *Overcoming Postnatal Depression: A Five Areas Approach* by C Williams, R Cantwell and K Robertson.
- *I'm Not Supposed to Feel Like This: A Christian Self-help Approach to Depression and Anxiety* by C Williams, P Richards and I Whitton.

Would you like something short and to the point? The following short, full-colour little CBT books by Dr Chris Williams are available from **www.fiveareas.com**:

- The Worry Box (a four-book set – Worry/panic, Face it, Fix it, Forget it)

Also:

- 1, 2, 3 Chill Relaxation CD (anxiety control training)
- Why do I feel so bad?
- How to fix almost everything
- Why does everything always go wrong?
- I can't be bothered doing anything
- Are you strong enough to keep your temper (anger)
- I'm not good enough (low confidence)

www.livinglifetothefull.com

This website offers free online training courses that teach key life skills by using the same model used in this book. There are useful additional handouts as well as DVD-based videos to learn key life skills confidentially and for free. You can download linked handouts as well as teaching exercises to reinforce and build on the changes you have made with the help of these course workbooks. It includes access to free MP3 relaxation downloads based on Anxiety Control Training.

Summary

In this workbook you have:

- Discovered what anxiety, worry and stress are.
- Understood how they can affect you.
- Identified the areas you need to tackle to overcome your own problems of anxiety.

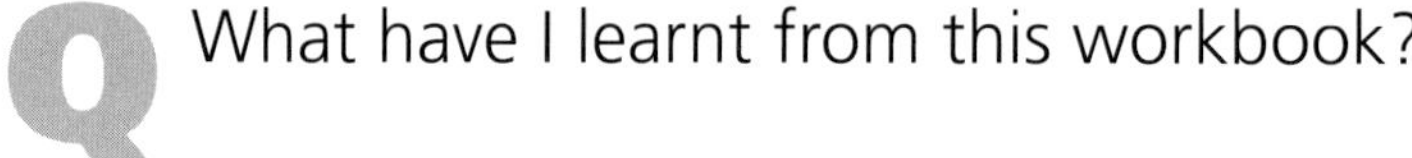

Q What have I learnt from this workbook?

Q What do I want to try *next*?

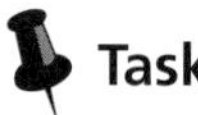

Task

Write down **three things** that went well every day for a week:

Stop, think and reflect on these points every evening. Why did these things go well? Use your answers to find out what are the helpful things you have done that you can build back into your life.

A request for feedback

An important part of the development of this course is that the content is updated on a regular basis, based on feedback from users and practitioners. Please send any feedback that you may have about this workbook to the address given below. You can also email your feedback. However, we can't answer specific questions or provide advice on treatment.

Address: Five Areas, PO Box 9, Glasgow G63 0WL, UK.

Our website: **www.livinglifetothefull.com**
email: **feedback@fiveareas.com**

My notes

My Anxiety diary

Date and time	Record your recent sleep/drink and feelings of pressure leading upto the anxiety	People and events leading up to feeling worse	My feelings at the time	My thoughts at the time	Altered physical symptoms	My altered behaviour
	When things improve also record what you were doing at the time they improved	– Where were you? – Who were you with? – What were you doing? – What was said/happened?	How were you feeling at the time? – Were you feeling anxious and panicky? – Any low mood? – Any other feelings (irritability, anger, guilt, shame)?	Any thoughts about: – Things not being fair? – Being picked on? – Being mocked/humiliated? – How you are coping? – The worst that could happen? – How others see you? – Your own body, behaviour or performance? – Any memories or mental pictures?	Note down any strong physical symptoms you noticed at the time, e.g. tense, rapid heartbeat, breaking out in a sweat, breathing faster, feeling shaky.	– What did you do differently? – What did you say differently – and how did you say it? – Did you stop doing what you were doing, or start doing something different? – Are you avoiding things because of how you feel? Please note down if you were overbreathing at the time (shallow, rapid breaths)

Overcoming Anxiety, Stress and Panic
A Five Areas Approach

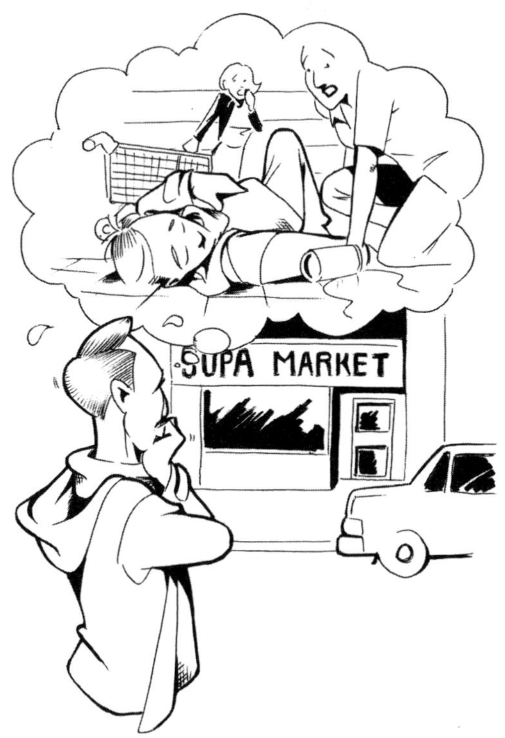

Understanding panic and phobias

www.livinglifetothefull.com
www.fiveareas.com

Dr Chris Williams

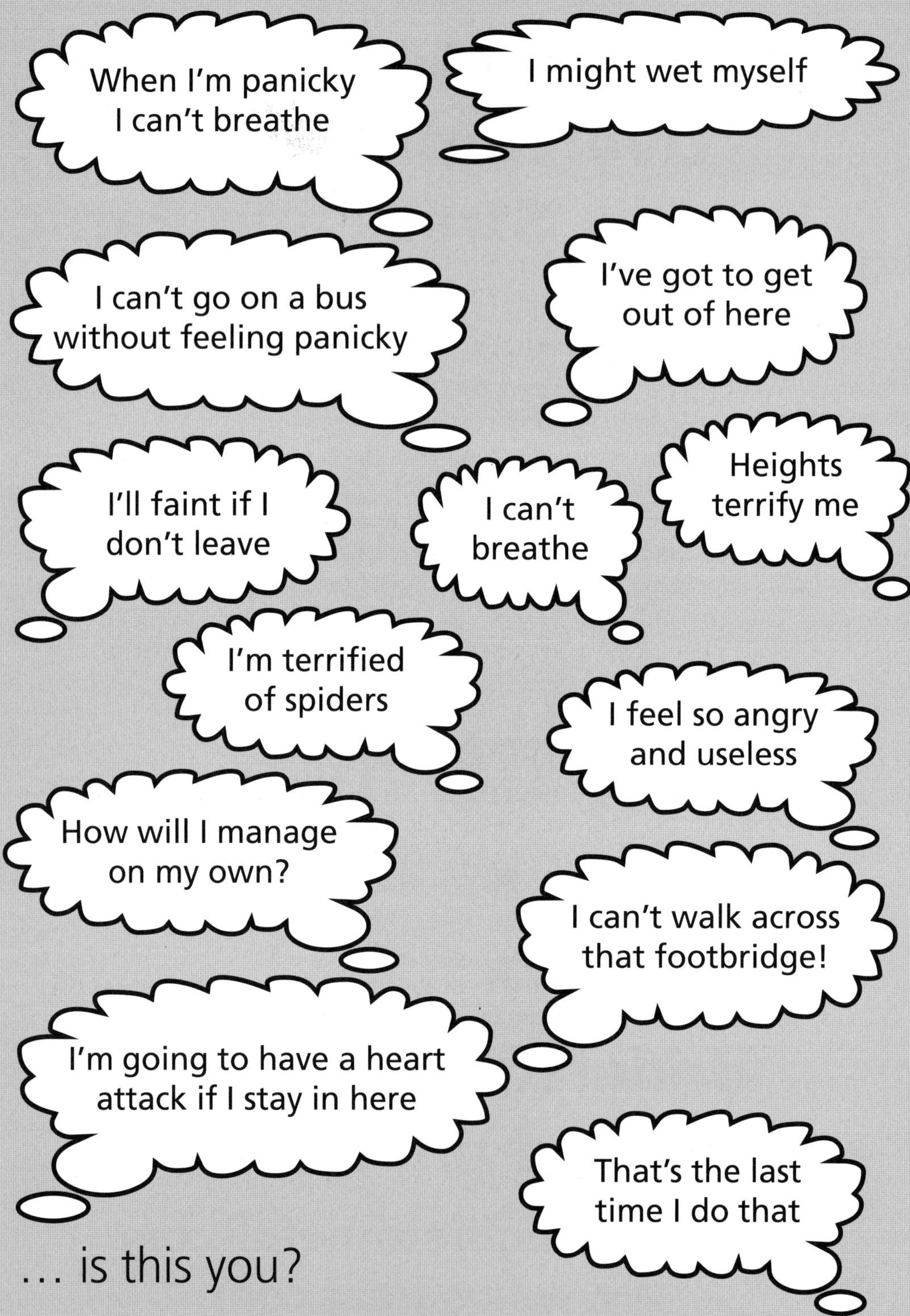
When I'm panicky I can't breathe
I might wet myself
I can't go on a bus without feeling panicky
I've got to get out of here
I'll faint if I don't leave
I can't breathe
Heights terrify me
I'm terrified of spiders
I feel so angry and useless
How will I manage on my own?
I can't walk across that footbridge!
I'm going to have a heart attack if I stay in here
That's the last time I do that

... is this you?

If it is ... this **workbook is for you**.

This workbook will help you to:

- Understand what panic and phobias are.
- Understand how they can affect you.
- Identify the areas you need to tackle to overcome your own problems of anxiety.

Understanding anxiety

Anxiety can affect everyone and anyone. Sometimes, anxiety can be helpful even though it can feel unpleasant. So for example, anxiety is helpful in situations of sudden danger, where it helps you to respond and get away as quickly as possible.

Anxiety becomes a problem when you feel extremely anxious in situations that are not dangerous at all. For example, being so anxious that you can't cross the road at a pedestrian crossing, or you can't enter a shop.

'Panic' is the word used to describe very high levels of anxiety and fear.

What is a panic attack?

Sometimes people become so anxious that they start to feel physically unwell. You feel terrified and stop what you are doing and try to leave or escape the situation. Or you may feel you can't move at all (paralysed – like the rabbit caught in the headlamps of a car) and freeze, expecting disaster to strike.

This feeling of terror is called a *panic attack*. A panic attack happens when there is a surge of adrenaline in your body (adrenaline is a hormone that your body produces that among other things makes your heart beat faster). This usually happens when you get scared. Because your body can produce only so much adrenaline, panic attacks rarely last longer than 20 to 30 minutes.

During a panic attack, you become convinced that something terrible or catastrophic is happening **right now**. Some common fears during a panic attack are:

- 'I'm going to faint.'
- 'I'm going to suffocate.'
- 'I'm going to collapse.'

- 'I'm going to have a stroke.'
- 'I'm going to have a heart attack.'

Sometimes the fear is of *going mad* or *losing control*. The main response is always to try to leave or escape.

Sometimes what starts as anxious worrying about problems can build up over time and turn into panic. Here is a checklist to help you recognise whether you are prone to panic attacks. As you are reading this workbook, you will probably have already gone through the checklist before in the *Tackling your anxiety: starting out (... and how to keep going if you feel stuck)* workbook. If you answered 'Yes' or 'Sometimes' to several of the questions in that checklist, then panic attacks are a problem for you.

Panic attack checklist

Q Do I notice anxiety that rises to a peak?

Yes ☐ No ☐ Sometimes ☐

Q Do I feel very scared and physically unwell during the panic attack?

Yes ☐ No ☐ Sometimes ☐

Q Do I fear that something terrible or catastrophic will happen during that time?

Yes ☐ No ☐ Sometimes ☐

Q Do I become overly aware of the things that I fear might happen during panic?

Yes ☐ No ☐ Sometimes ☐

Q Do I stop what I am doing and try to immediately escape or leave when I feel like this?

Yes ☐ No ☐ Sometimes ☐

Q Am I downplaying my own ability to overcome these problems?

Yes ☐ No ☐ Sometimes ☐

If you have answered 'Yes' or 'Sometimes' to any of these questions, then panic may be a problem for you.

How common is panic?

You may be surprised to learn that about one in 20 people have panic attacks at any one time. So besides you, at least one or two more people in your street might also be having problems with panic. There will also be people who have had problems with panic in the past.

Panic attacks often occur as part of other mental health problems, especially depression, worries and phobias.

Let's find out more about phobias.

What is a phobia?

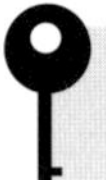

Key point

A *phobia* means having high levels of anxiety (often with panic attacks) regularly in a particular situation. You become overly aware of any possible threats linked to the fear. So you try to avoid or quickly leave the situation that causes you to feel anxious. People often know logically that the situation will not harm or kill them, yet they get anxious anyway.

Here is a checklist (again repeated from the *Tackling your anxiety: starting out (… and how to keep going if you feel stuck)* workbook to help you recognise whether you may have a phobia.

Phobia checklist

Q Do I feel very anxious or do I panic when I face particular situations, people or places?

Yes ☐ No ☐ Sometimes ☐

Q Does even thinking about these situations/places/people make me feel nervous?

Yes ☐ No ☐ Sometimes ☐

Q Have I become too sensitive to anything to do with the phobic fear?

Yes ☐ No ☐ Sometimes ☐

Q Am I downplaying my own ability to overcome these fears?

Yes ☐ No ☐ Sometimes ☐

Q Am I avoiding these situations, places or people?

Yes ☐ No ☐ Sometimes ☐

Q Overall, is my life becoming increasingly restricted as a result?

Yes ☐ No ☐ Sometimes ☐

If you have answered 'Yes' or 'Sometimes' to any of these questions, then you may have a phobia.

How did things get to be like this?

The first step of working out how to change things like having panic attacks or a phobia is to understand how things have come to this. You can use a time line to find out how you started to feel this way. An example is shown below.

Example: Harvinder's time line

- Beginning:

  March: I had a lot on at work and home. One day when I was out shopping, I suddenly felt very hot and faint. I had to go home.

  End of March: Had a full panic attack – felt hot, dizzy and scared I might suffocate.

  April: I was struggling to cope and lying awake worrying about how I was going to get everything done. Started to get scared going into large, busy shops or on buses where I couldn't get off. Started avoiding these and only going to the local corner shop.

  June: I went off work sick because it was too hard to get there on the bus.

  August: I was due to return to work this month. But my GP is suggesting that I should see a mental health practitioner. I'm still very scared going to the shops and I'm avoiding buses completely.

- Today:

  I have started using the course workbooks – I want to find out what's causing me to feel like this.

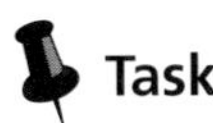 **Task**

Now it's your turn. Fill in your own time line below.

Beginning (a time when I didn't get panic attacks or didn't have a phobia):

Today:

The good news is that your time line doesn't stop here. If you can make changes, you can move forwards and feel better again.

So the next step then is to see how panic or a phobia is affecting you.

Understanding how you feel using the Five Areas Approach

One helpful way of understanding how panic and phobias affect you is to think of the ways that these conditions affect the different areas of your life. The **Five Areas Approach** can help you to do this by looking in detail at five important areas of your life.

The Five Areas are:

- **Area 1: The people and events around you**. This includes the situations you face and people or places you find particularly hard to cope with.
- **Area 2: Your thinking**. This can often become extreme and unhelpful when you panic or when you have a phobia. Scary thoughts can cause you to jump to the very worst conclusions.
- **Area 3: Your feelings (also called moods or emotions)**. You can feel tense, scared or irritable when you are phobic or feeling panicky.
- **Area 4: Any altered physical symptoms in your body**.
- **Area 5: Your altered behaviour or activity levels**. This includes both – the helpful things you can do to make you feel better, and the unhelpful things you do, which backfire and make you feel even worse.

Try to think about how the Five Areas assessment can help Harvinder understand how he is feeling.

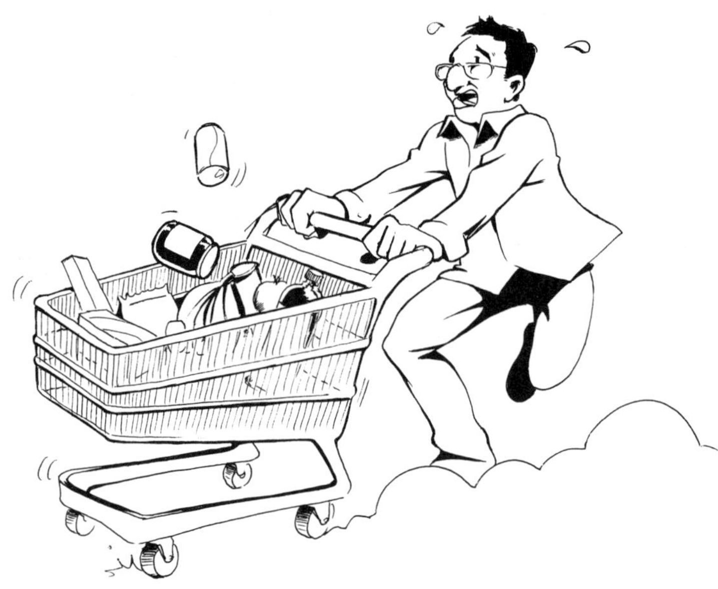

Example: How panic attacks are affecting Harvinder's life

Harvinder has started to feel anxious and panicky whenever he goes to the supermarket. He has avoided going there as much as he can, using local shops more instead. Although his avoidance has helped him feel less anxious, it's now affecting his life as he needs to go to a larger shop for some things.

On the way to the supermarket he is very aware of his heart thumping. As he enters the store his breathing speeds right up and his heart starts racing. He fears that he will pass out and collapse. As he breathes faster and faster he starts to feel dizzy and spaced out. He tries to cope and make himself feel better by:

- Trying desperately hard not to think about how he feels.
- Walking faster than usual, holding tightly to the shopping trolley.
- Trying to control his breathing by taking rapid breaths. This makes things worse.
- Escaping/leaving when he feels bad: after only five minutes he abandons the trolley in the middle of the store and walks/runs outside.
- He pledges that he will never go back into another supermarket.

Leaving the supermarket helps him feel safer in the short term. However, in the longer term, his avoidance backfires and undermines his confidence.

Harvinder felt ill because of his anxious overbreathing and the adrenaline surge in his body. However, high anxiety isn't dangerous. If Harvinder had stayed put inside the supermarket his symptoms would have settled down. Staying inside would have allowed him to test out if his fear of collapsing would really happen. He would have discovered that the worst would not occur, and over time (20 to 40 minutes) he would have felt better.

By leaving the shop, Harvinder increased his fears that it was dangerous staying and he could only cope by leaving. He then promises himself never to visit a supermarket again.

The figure below shows how Harvinder's problems can be summarised using the Five Areas Approach.

Harvinder's Five Areas summary

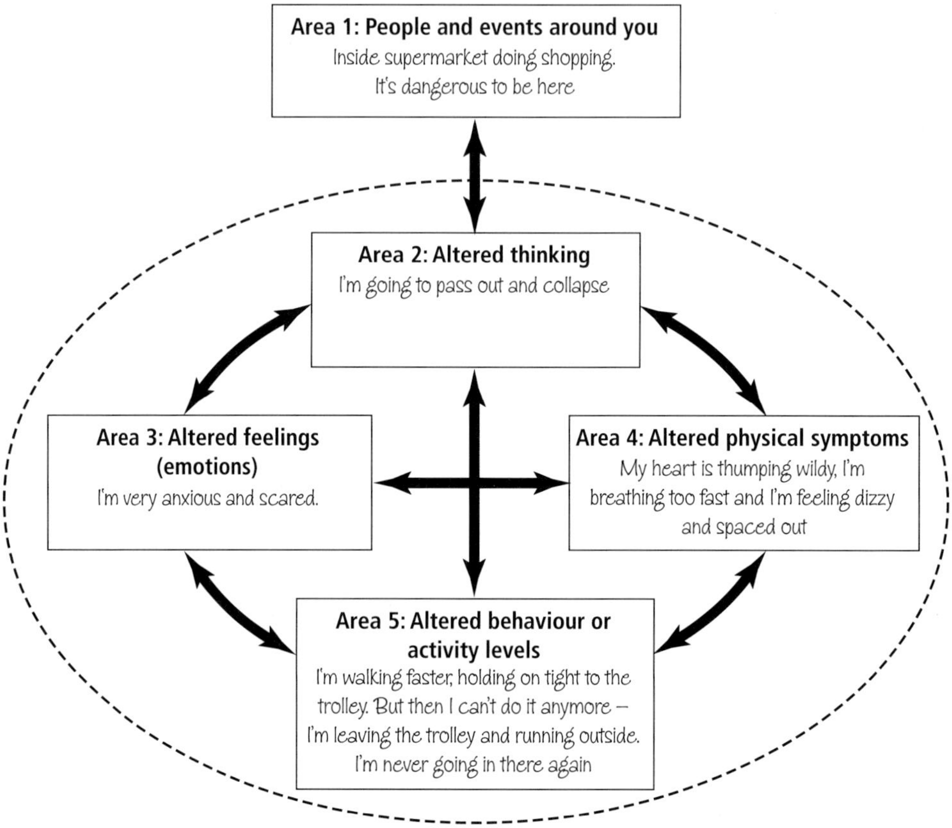

Area 1: People and events around you
Inside supermarket doing shopping.
It's dangerous to be here

Area 2: Altered thinking
I'm going to pass out and collapse

Area 3: Altered feelings (emotions)
I'm very anxious and scared.

Area 4: Altered physical symptoms
My heart is thumping wildy, I'm breathing too fast and I'm feeling dizzy and spaced out

Area 5: Altered behaviour or activity levels
I'm walking faster, holding on tight to the trolley. But then I can't do it anymore – I'm leaving the trolley and running outside. I'm never going in there again

The Five Areas diagram shows that what you think about a situation or problem can affect how you feel physically and emotionally. It also shows that your thinking affects what you do (your behaviour or activity levels). Look at the arrows in the diagram. Each of the Five Areas of your life affect each other.

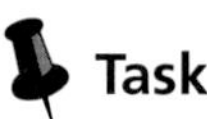

Task

Let's take a look at what's happening for you in each of the Five Areas, starting with Area 1.

Area 1: People and events around you

All of us from time to time face practical problems such as:

- Facing up to people, places and events that scare us.
- Problems with family and life at home.
- Problems in relationships with partners, friends or colleagues.
- Other life challenges, for example work that needs to be done, time pressures, having too many things on at once, problems at work, college, etc.

Are any of these relevant to you?

- There is no one around who I can really talk to.

  Yes ☐ No ☐ Sometimes ☐

- I am struggling to cope with my work.

  Yes ☐ No ☐ Sometimes ☐

- My baby isn't feeding/sleeping easily.

  Yes ☐ No ☐ Sometimes ☐

- I worry about work or money or debts.

  Yes ☐ No ☐ Sometimes ☐

- There are problems where I live.

  Yes ☐ No ☐ Sometimes ☐

- My children won't do what I tell them.

  Yes ☐ No ☐ Sometimes ☐

- It's hard to get on with another person or people in my family.

  Yes ☐ No ☐ Sometimes ☐

- I am having problems with my neighbours.

  Yes ☐ No ☐ Sometimes ☐

- I have problems with colleagues at work.

  Yes ☐ No ☐ Sometimes ☐

- I/My family has unemployment worries.

  Yes ☐ No ☐ Sometimes ☐

- I/My family has housing problems.

  Yes ☐ No ☐ Sometimes ☐

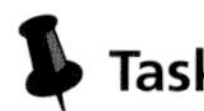

Task

Now make a list of any other problems you face. You may also find it helpful to write in some more detail about any of the problems you noted in the list above. Use an extra sheet of paper if you need to, or use the **My Notes** section at the end of this workbook.

Summary for Area 1: People and events around you

Now rate the extent of your problems in this area.

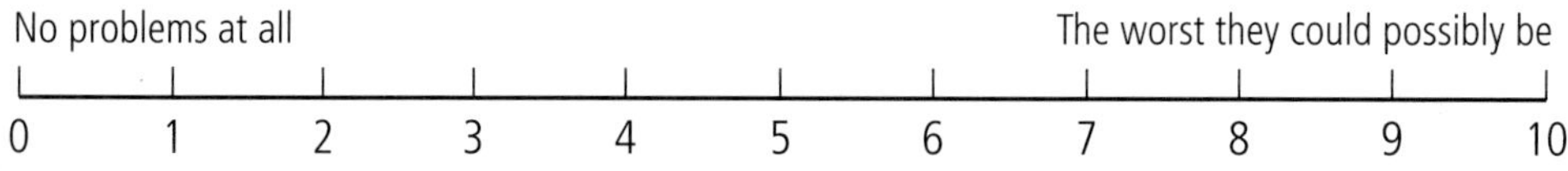

What next?

Looking at your score, check whether the people and events around you (your situation) is an area you wish to work on. If you do, two of the workbooks in the course will help you to make changes in this area:

- *How to ask for what you really need (being assertive)* – this workbook deals with how to be assertive and help you to rebalance your relationships.
- *How to start fixing problems and finding solutions (practical problem solving).*

Area 2: Your thinking

When someone feels anxious, panicky or phobic, how they **think** tends to change.

Your thinking becomes:

- Extreme.
- Unhelpful.
- Catastrophic – so that you believe the very worst will happen and that you cannot cope.

As explained before in this workbook, what you think can affect how you are. Let's look at how Sam notices this below.

Example: How Sam's thinking can affect how she feels and what she does

Some people get very anxious when others are watching them perform a task, such as giving a talk or doing karaoke. Any other situation where the person is the centre of attention can cause similar symptoms. For example, Sam is a teacher and becomes very anxious leading a class. She fears that 'I'll mess it up', 'I'll stumble over the words', 'My head-teacher will find me out', and that 'the pupils will laugh and I'll lose all credibility'. The fears go round and round in her head and the anxiety builds up and up.

So every time before going into class, Sam begins to tense up, and feels overly hot and sweaty. She begins to feel increasingly panicky. She keeps dabbing at her brow (an action designed to make her feel safer) and talks far faster to get through it all. She eventually decides to cut the talk short (avoidance). She asks the children to do a computer-based task while she asks a secretary to get a teaching colleague to relieve her. She lies down in the staff room and goes home early saying she thinks she has caught 'a bug'. At home she starts crying – worrying whether her days as a teacher are over. This avoidance increases her fear that she can't do her job any more.

The table below shows how Sam's and two more people's thoughts, feelings and behaviours affect each other.

People and events around us	Altered thinking	Unhelpful thinking style (s)	Altered Emotional and/or physical impact	Altered Behaviour change
Sam is about to do a talk for her class	I'll mess it up I'll stumble over the words The pupils will laugh and I'll lose all credibility	Catastrophic thinking and not believing she can cope Mind reading	Feels very anxious, physically tense and sweaty	*Avoidance*: Sam cuts the teaching short and goes home thinking she's ill *Unhelpful behaviours*: Sam talks quickly and keeps dabbing her forehead with a handkerchief
Jane is sitting in her main room when suddenly a spider runs across the carpet	It's horrible, it will bite me. I can't deal with this	Catastrophic thinking and not believing she can cope	Anxious, embarrassed and feels physically tense.	*Avoidance*: Jane jumps on to the settee and then runs away *Unhelpful behaviours*: asks neighbour to remove the spider, and repeatedly checks that she has done so.
Harvinder has had fears of going shopping for over six months and these are gradually getting worse. He is now in the middle of a long queue at the supermarket	I'm going to collapse and pass out	Catastrophic thinking and not believing he can cope	Anxiety and physical symptoms of a faster heart rate and rapid breathing	*Avoidance*: Harvinder is tending to avoid supermarkets, and only shopping there when it is quieter *Unhelpful behaviours*: Harvinder leaves the queue and walks round the store faster than usual, gripping tightly to the trolley. But then he abandons the trolley and quickly leaves the store

During a panic attack, people feel strongly that something terrible is happening right then. You may **jump to the very worst conclusion** (catastrophic thinking) that things will go very badly wrong. You may overlook your own strengths and be very self-critical. Overall, your thinking becomes extreme, unhelpful and out of all proportion. Your own strengths and ability to cope are overlooked or downplayed. Things then seem as if they are out of control.

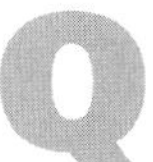

Do you notice any of the common catastrophic thoughts listed below when you are panicking?

Catastrophic thought	Tick here if you notice this thought sometimes when you panic
'I'm going to faint or collapse/pass out.'	☐
'I'm going to suffocate.'	☐
'I'm going to collapse.'	☐
'I'm going to have a stroke.'	☐
'I'm going to have a heart attack.'	☐
'I'm going to wet or poo myself.'	☐
'I'm going to go mad.'	☐
'I'm going to lose control.'	☐
'I'm going to show myself up/make a fool of myself.'	☐
'I can't cope with this'	☐

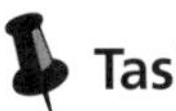

Task

Write any other catastrophic fears you have here:

Images and mental pictures – an important part of anxiety

Sometimes people notice mental pictures or images in their mind when they become anxious. Images are a form of thought. They may be 'still' images (for example, a photograph) or moving images (for example, a video). Images may be in black and white or be in colour. They may include a mental picture of some catastrophic event occurring, such as collapsing, suffocating, or of your own funeral. As with all anxious fears, the images add to your feelings of anxiety.

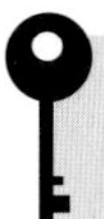

Key point

High levels of anxiety are unpleasant but not dangerous.

Remember that each of the Five Areas can affect each other. Your bodily reactions can therefore worsen (reinforce) your fears. So, fears of having a heart attack or stroke are reinforced when you notice altered physical feelings caused by the panic. So, a feeling of tightness in your chest or a rapidly beating heart can convince you that you are having a heart attack. Similarly, feelings of dizziness (because of anxious overbreathing) can worsen the fears of having a stroke or collapsing.

Summary for Area 2: Your thinking

Rate the extent of your problems in this area.

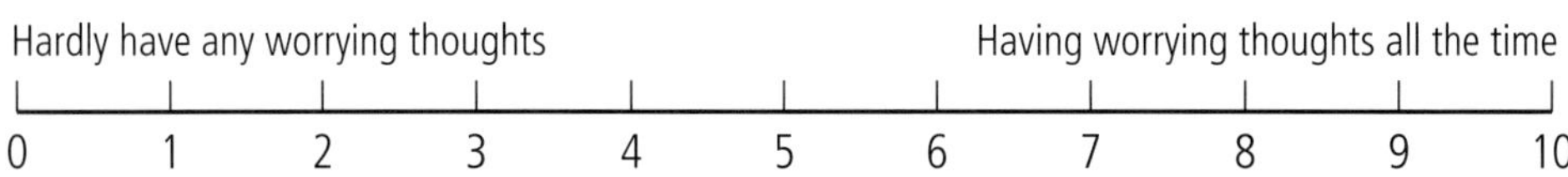

What next?

If this is an area you wish to work on, the *Noticing and changing anxious thinking* workbook will help you to find out more and change these ways of thinking.

Area 3: Your feelings (emotions)

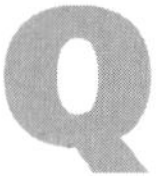

What emotional changes have you noticed over the past two weeks?

- Worry, stress or tension?

  Yes ☐ No ☐ Sometimes ☐

- High levels of anxiety or panic (panic attacks)?

  Yes ☐ No ☐ Sometimes ☐

- Lowness or sadness?

  Yes ☐ No ☐ Sometimes ☐

- Reduced or no sense of pleasure in things?

  Yes ☐ No ☐ Sometimes ☐

- Loss of all feelings, for example, noticing no feelings at all?

  Yes ☐ No ☐ Sometimes ☐

- Guilt?

  Yes ☐ No ☐ Sometimes ☐

- Anger or irritability (common if you are trying to escape during panic)?

  Yes ☐ No ☐ Sometimes ☐

- Shame or embarrassment?

  Yes ☐ No ☐ Sometimes ☐

- Other changes in how you feel (write down here):

Your feelings (emotions) are an important and normal part of your life. Changes in how you feel are often linked with your thoughts, memories and the ideas that are going through your mind at the time. Try to become aware of these thoughts and note them down when there is a change in how you feel.

The good news is that by noticing these changes you can begin to slowly make helpful changes in how you feel.

Depersonalisation: feeling cut-off and disconnected from things

Panic and high anxiety can make us feel mentally disconnected and cut-off from things. Healthcare professionals call this *depersonalisation*. It can sometimes be difficult to describe exactly what this feels like. Many people notice a *fuzzy-headed*, *spaced-out* sort of feeling. You may know that you are fully awake and also exactly where you are. Yet in spite of this you feel far away from things – as if you are a robot functioning on automatic.

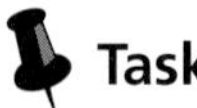

Task

If you would like to find out more about depersonalisation, read the *Understanding and overcoming feelings of depersonalisation* workbook.

Summary for Area 3: Your feelings (emotions)

Having been through the emotions checklist above, rate the extent of your problems in this area on the graph below.

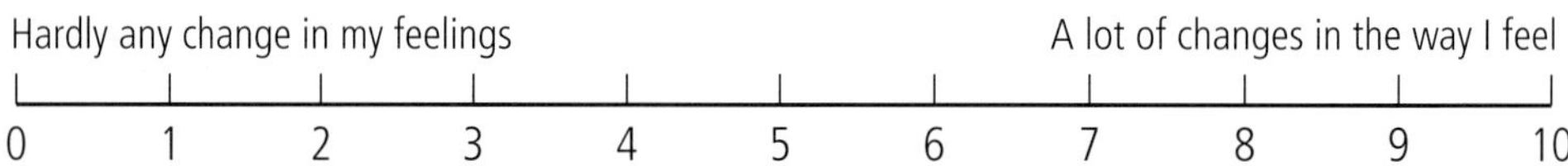

What next?

If this is an area you wish to work on, by making helpful changes in any of the other four areas, you can change how you feel in a positive way.

Area 4: Altered physical symptoms

When a person becomes very anxious and panicky, they notice a variety of physical changes.

Which of the following physical symptoms have you noticed when you feel panicky?

- Do you have a dry mouth?

Yes ☐ No ☐ Sometimes ☐

- Do you breathe too quickly, with rapid shallow breaths?

Yes ☐ No ☐ Sometimes ☐

- Do you notice a rapid or thumping heart?

Yes ☐ No ☐ Sometimes ☐

- Do you have a fuzzy-headed or faint feeling, or headaches?

  Yes ☐ No ☐ Sometimes ☐

- Do your muscles get tense or do you feel restless or on edge (fidgety)?

  Yes ☐ No ☐ Sometimes ☐

- Do you feel shaky, hot, clammy or cold?

  Yes ☐ No ☐ Sometimes ☐

- Do you notice butterflies or a churning feeling in your stomach, or do you feel sick or want to go to the toilet frequently?

  Yes ☐ No ☐ Sometimes ☐

- Do you get pain, for example a painful chest, tummy or headaches – as if your head is in a vice or might explode?

  Yes ☐ No ☐ Sometimes ☐

- Do you notice a strong urge to wee or poo?

  Yes ☐ No ☐ Sometimes ☐

- Do you not feel like having sex or worry about your performance?

  Yes ☐ No ☐ Sometimes ☐

- Do you have any other symptoms?

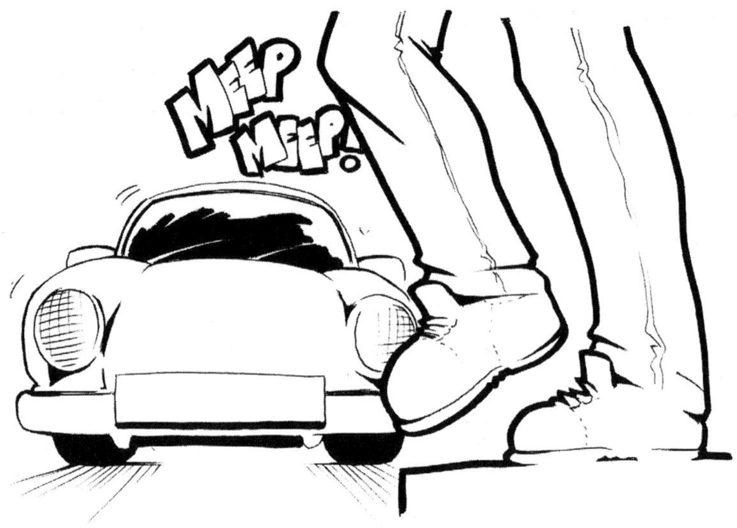

What causes these physical symptoms?

Your body reacts to frightening thoughts just as it would to a physical danger. The **fight or flight adrenaline response** creates all of the symptoms described above. Your heart rate and breathing both speed up so that your muscles are ready to react to defend yourself or run away. This is very useful when the danger is real. Think about a time when you have had a sudden shock – perhaps being chased by a barking dog. Your body produces adrenaline, which makes your heart beat faster. There may be other physical responses such as feeling sweaty or restless and tense. Breathing may speed up to allow more oxygen to get to the muscles. Sometimes rapid breathing continues long enough to cause a condition of anxious overbreathing – this is also called *hyperventilation*.

Summary for Area 4: Altered physical symptoms

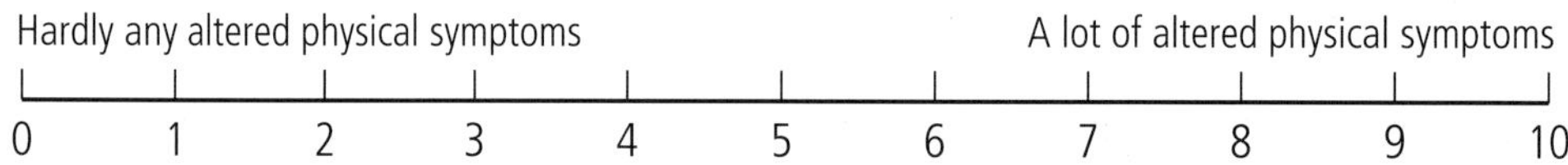

Having answered the questions, rate the extent of your problems in this graph.

What next?

The good news is that by making changes in other areas, you can improve how you feel physically. You will find some helpful advice about how to tackle many of your physical symptoms or feelings in the *Overcoming anxious overbreathing (hyperventilation)* workbook. You can also learn a relaxation technique such as Anxiety Control Training by downloading three recordings from **www.fiveareas.com**.

Area 5: Altered behaviour or activity levels

You have already worked hard in thinking about the first four of the five areas in your Five Areas Assessment – well done! Here you look at the last area – altered behaviour (things that you do).

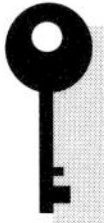

Key point

Making changes in your behaviour and activity levels are some of the most helpful things you can do to boost how you feel.

Some things that you do can worsen how you feel. On the other hand, many ways in which you respond can be very helpful and boost how you are feeling. The ways in which your altered behaviours may worsen things are:

First type of altered behaviour: Reduced activity

When you feel stressed, tense or down, it's hard to keep doing things because you have:

- Low energy and feel tired ('I'm too tired').
- Little enjoyment or achievement when you do things.
- Negative thoughts about things ('I just can't be bothered').

All these lead to reduced activity – where you do less of or stop doing things **which are important** to you. Often the first things that are squeezed out are things that have previously given you a sense of **fun** or **achievement** (for example, meeting up with friends, and doing things with your family). You can also lose your sense of **closeness** to others.

It begins to feel as though everything is too much effort. And so you feel worse and worse.

Write down any examples of reduced activity you have noticed here:

The good news is that once you have noticed whether this is true for you, you can start working on your reduced activity in a planned, step-by-step way. You will find some suggestions for how to do this in the workbook *Facing fears and overcoming avoidance*.

Second type of altered behaviour: Avoiding or escaping from things

People often start to avoid or escape from people, places and situations that make them feel stressed. This may make you feel less anxious in the short term. But in the longer term, avoiding things makes it harder and harder to confidently face your fears in the future. And you don't see that your worst fears don't actually occur. In fact, avoidance teaches people the unhelpful rule that you only coped with a situation by avoiding it.

Key point

Avoidance and escaping can make you feel worse and also undermine your confidence.

Some things you may be avoiding

- Heights or places where you could fall.
- Insects such as spiders, bees, moths, flies, butterflies or wasps.
- Enclosed spaces where you can feel trapped in your seat such as buses, trains, aeroplanes, cinemas or theatres.
- Going shopping in supermarkets or shopping arcades, etc.
- Talking about how anxious and scared you are feeling.

Write down some examples of activities or things you have been avoiding here:

The good news is that once you have noticed that you are tending to avoid things, you can start working on tackling avoidance and escaping. You need to do this in a planned, step-by-step way. The workbook *Facing fears and overcoming avoidance* tells you how to do this.

Third type of altered behaviour: Dropping helpful things you do

Helpful behaviours include doing things such as:

- Talking to friends or family for support.
- Recognising the times when you have been too hard on yourself.
- Reading or using self-help materials, or attending a self-help group.
- Going to see a doctor or healthcare practitioner.
- Finding activities or meeting people who give you a boost.
- If you have a personal spiritual faith, your beliefs may provide helpful support.

My helpful behaviours

Q Has the anxiety, phobia or panic caused you to stop doing activities that help you?

Yes ☐ No ☐ Sometimes ☐

Write down any examples of helpful things you do here:

It is important to make time to keep doing these activities as they really do help.

Fourth type of altered behaviour: Unhelpful things you do

Sometimes people may do things that make them feel better at first but, in the longer term, these things backfire and make you feel worse. Do you do any of the following unhelpful behaviours?

Trying to escape and hurry away:

- Rushing through a task so you can leave quickly.
- Walking more quickly than normal.
- Making an excuse, or lying and saying you are ill or have another urgent reason why you need to leave early or not attend.
- Quickly leaving a place or situation when you feel bad.

Distracting yourself mentally by trying hard not to think about how you feel. For example:

- Trying desperately hard not to think about how you feel.
- Trying to block how you feel by doing things that make you feel safer *mentally* (like doing maths sums or saying 'I'm all right' again and again or focusing on the lines on the floor) or through *actions* (such as biting your lip or digging your nails into your hand, gripping hard onto things for support etc).

Blocking how you feel using other approaches:

- Using alcohol or street drugs to block how you feel.
- Misusing prescribed medication by taking extra doses that are not prescribed to block how you feel.
- Asking someone to accompany you if you feel scared.
- Seeking reassurance from others all the time.

Other unhelpful behaviours are:

- Withdrawing into yourself and cutting yourself off from your friends or family.
- Neglecting yourself (for example, by not eating as much or not washing).
- Finding yourself tempted to do things that you know are unwise or wrong. This might include deliberately taking risks, picking fights or betraying a partner.
- Harming yourself as a way of blocking how you feel (for example, self-cutting).
- Shouting or screaming at others out of frustration or getting angry if people seem to crowd you or push you when you are panicking.

Write down any examples of unhelpful behaviour you do here:

The purpose of all the unhelpful behaviours is to feel safer/better, at least in the short term. Therefore, they are sometimes called *safety behaviours*. But, although safety behaviours may help you feel better in the short term, this doesn't last. **The anxiety returns to the same or an even higher level.** For example, drinking too much alcohol or taking sedative drugs may give you a sense of false courage, but such things lead to more problems of their own.

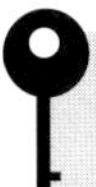

Key point

An important thing to watch out for is whether you have got into a habit of reacting to difficult situations in certain ways. By watching out for any unhelpful behaviours that you fall into, and by choosing to respond differently, you can make large changes in how you are feeling.

You will find out more about reducing unhelpful behaviours in the workbook *Things you do that worsen your anxiety (unhelpful behaviours)*.

Summary for Area 5: Any altered behaviours or activity levels

Now think about all the altered behaviours you have identified and rate the extent of your problems in this area.

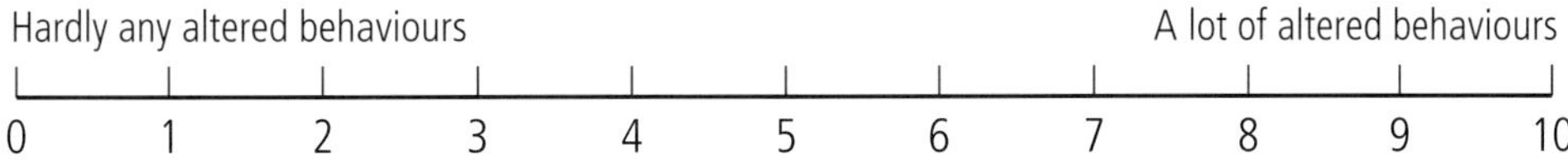

What next?

Remember that the purpose of the Five Areas Approach is to help you recognise how your panicking or phobia is affecting you. This can help you decide which areas you need to work on to bring about change.

The good news is that all the areas are linked so that making changes in any one area can lead to change in the others. So if you try to alter any one of these areas, it will help you tackle your problem.

Spotting patterns that affect your panic response or your phobia

The first thing is to do some research on how you feel.

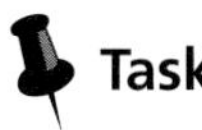

Task

Use the Anxiety diary at the end of the workbook to record **all the times** when you are feeling panicky or phobic over the next week. You can download more pages for free from **www.fiveareas.com**. The aim is to play detective and identify the things that are worsening the situation for you.

Then write down what you discover.

What seems to make it worse or better?

- Do you panic more first thing in the morning? (This could mean you have depression or you are sleeping poorly.)

- Do certain situations seem to affect how bad your panic or phobia gets? (For example, is it affected by stressful, or particular, situations such as crowds, heights or supermarkets?)

- Do certain other feelings seem to affect how bad your panic or phobia gets? (For example, is it affected by feeling low or anxious, angry, guilty or ashamed?)

- Does thinking too much or worrying about particular fears make your panicking or phobia worse?

- Does poor sleep or rapid breathing affect how you feel?

- Does doing exercise make your panic feel better?

- If you are using any medication, alcohol or street drugs, do you feel worse within a couple of hours of using them?

Identifying your early warning signs

Use your Anxiety diary to think back in detail about some of the recent times when you have panicked. Were there any early warning signs:

- Either that some of the things that bring on the panic were building up?
- Or that you were beginning to become panicky?

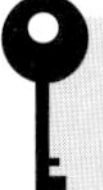

Key point

Early warning signs of panic include:

- Altered thinking: with scared, anxious or very depressing worries.
- Altered feelings: for example, with rising tension and fear, dropping mood or becoming irritated or angry.
- Altered physical symptoms: for example, getting hot, sweaty, fidgety, noticing more rapid breathing or heart rate, or muscle tenseness.
- Altered behaviour or activity levels: for example, drinking more, walking faster, trying to get out of a situation, raising your voice, rushing away, pushing people or being rude to escape a scary situation, or trying to avoid things such as conversations.

By noticing these key early warning signs you can **do something about it** – before it worsens to become a panic attack or a phobia.

Making changes

Use your answers to the questions above to work out what longer-term changes you need to make in your life. The good news is that you can learn to do something different when you start to feel panicky or phobic.

Where do you start?

The workbooks in this course can help you begin to tackle all of the five problem areas of anxiety, panic and phobias.

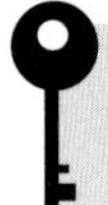

Key point

One key to success is to try **not to tackle everything at once**. You are more likely to improve by taking slow, steady steps. If you are too enthusiastic at the start and try to change too much together, you can run out of steam. So try to take things one step at a time by choosing and focusing on a particular area you are going to start with.

Set yourself:

- Short-term targets: these are changes you can make today, tomorrow and next week.
- Medium-term targets: these are changes to be put in place over the next few weeks.
- Long-term targets: this is where you want to be in six months or a year.

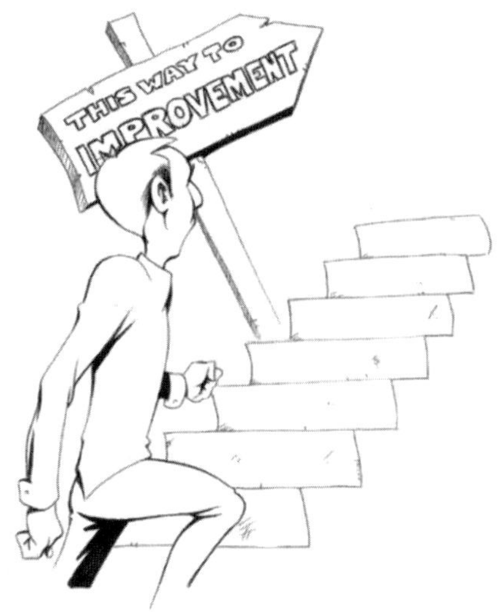

Which workbook should you try first?

Your Five Areas assessment will help you choose which area to work on and which workbook to read first. This means that you are actively choosing not to focus on the other areas to start with.

Because all of the Five Areas of your life affect each other, choosing any of the areas to start on makes sense. Just choose something **you** want to work on now.

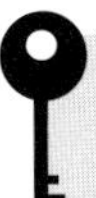

Key point

There isn't a set 'course' in this book. The course you take will include as many workbooks as you feel you need to use.

In the table below, put a tick next to the workbooks you plan to read and also put a tick after you have completed it. Put a * by the first workbook you will work on.

Repeat your **Five Areas assessment** after using each workbook to help you decide where to go next.

How do I know if I need extra help?

Ideally, people using these workbooks will have someone to support doing it. But there are times when this won't be enough. If you struggle to do the tasks in the workbooks don't worry. Just do what you can. But if things *still* do not seem to be improving, you may need to get extra help.

If you have somebody supporting you, discuss what you have been doing with them. Otherwise make an appointment to see your doctor or a mental health worker.

Workbook	Plan to read	Tick when completed
Understanding why you feel as you do		
Tackling your anxiety: starting out (... and how to keep going if you feel stuck)	☐	☐
Understanding worry and stress	☐	☐
Understanding panic and phobias	☐	☐
Making changes to do with people and events around us		
How to start fixing problems and finding solutions (practical problem solving)	☐	☐
How to ask for what you really need (being assertive)	☐	☐
Learning to be calmer, less annoyed and less irritated	☐	☐
Making changes in your life		
How to get a good night's sleep: overcoming anxiety and sleep problems	☐	☐
Using exercise to overcome stress	☐	☐
Things you do that worsen your anxiety (unhelpful behaviours)	☐	☐
Stress, alcohol and drugs	☐	☐
Facing fears and overcoming avoidance	☐	☐
Understanding and overcoming shyness and social phobia	☐	☐
Noticing and changing anxious thinking	☐	☐
Understanding and overcoming feelings of depersonalisation	☐	☐
Overcoming anxious overbreathing (hyperventilation)	☐	☐

Two additional workbooks, *Understanding and using anti-anxiety medication* and *Planning for the future* are available free from **www.livinglifetothefull.com**.

Sources of extra help

- **Your family doctor or GP**. Your GP can offer medical advice and (if they feel it is necessary) refer you to a mental health specialist for a detailed assessment.
- **Social services**. Social services can be a great source of support for families. You can find your local social services office hours enquiry phone number and a 24-hour emergency phone number in the *Yellow Pages*.

Other organisations you can approach are:

- Anxiety UK: this charity has excellent online resources at **www.anxietyuk.org.uk**. There are forums and live chat as well as email support. The charity also has a helpline (**08444 775 774** – Monday to Friday 9.30 am–5.30 pm).
- Triumph over Phobia: this charity runs local groups for people with anxiety, panic and obsessive-compulsive problems. (See **www.topuk.org** or call **0845 600 9601** or email: **info@topuk.org**).
- No Panic Web: this organisation offers telephone-based support, classes and mentoring. (See **www.nopanic.org.uk**; telephone help line in the UK: **0808 808 0545**; outside the UK: **0044 1 952 590 545**; in Ireland: **01 272 1897**.)
- Royal College of Psychiatrists: you can get fact sheets about panic and phobias from the college's website (**www.rcpsych.ac.uk**) or by calling **020 7235 2351**.
- British Association for Behavioural and Cognitive Psychotherapies: the website of this organisation (**www.babcp.com**) has information about cognitive behavioural therapy and a list of accredited cognitive behaviour therapy practitioners and how to access them.

Other books that may be of help

You can buy the following helpful books from local or online bookshops including **www.fiveareas.com/books**, or you may find them at your local library:

- *Overcoming Depression and Low Mood: A Five Areas Approach*, third edition by C Williams.
- *Overcoming Teenage Depression and Low Mood: A Five Areas Approach* by N Dummett and C Williams.

- *Overcoming Postnatal Depression: A Five Areas Approach* by C Williams, R Cantwell and K Robertson.
- *I'm Not Supposed to Feel Like This: A Christian Self-help Approach to Depression and Anxiety* by C Williams, P Richards and I Whitton.

Would you like something short and to the point?

The following short, key, full colour books by Dr Chris Williams are available from **www.fiveareas.com**:

- The Worry Box (a four-book set – Worry/panic, Face it, Fix it, Forget it)
- Why do I feel so bad?
- Why does everything always go wrong?
- Are you strong enough to keep your temper (anger)
- I'm not good enough (low confidence)
- 10 things you can do to make you feel happier straight away

... and others available from **www.fiveareas.com**.

www.livinglifetothefull.com

This website offers free online training courses that teach key life skills by using the same model used in this book. There are useful additional handouts as well as DVD-based videos to learn key life skills confidentially and for free. You can download linked handouts as well as teaching exercises to reinforce and build on the changes you have made with the help of these course workbooks. It includes access to free MP3 relaxation downloads based on Anxiety Control Training.

Summary

In this workbook you have:

- Understood what panic and phobias are.
- Found out how they can affect you.

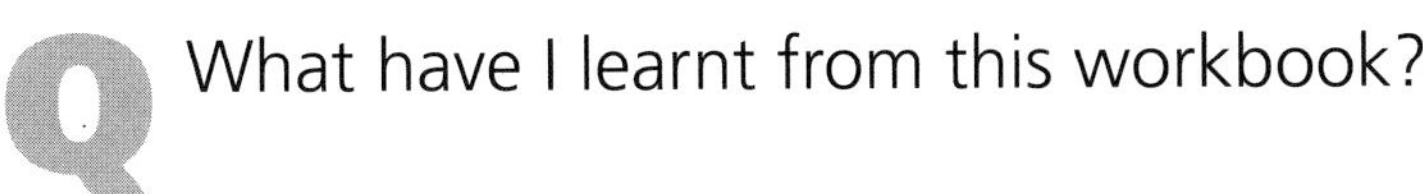

What have I learnt from this workbook?

What do I want to try *next*?

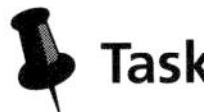

Task

Write down **three things** that went well every day for a week:

Stop, think and reflect on these points every evening. Why did these things go well?

Use these things to find out what are the helpful things you have done that you can build back into your life.

A request for feedback

An important part of the development of this course is that the content is updated on a regular basis, based on feedback from users and practitioners. Please send any feedback that you may have about this workbook to the address given below. You can also email your feedback. However, we can't answer specific questions or provide advice on treatment.

Address: Five Areas, PO Box 9, Glasgow G63 0WL, UK.

Our website: **www.livinglifetothefull.com**
email: **feedback@fiveareas.com**

My notes

PART 2

Making changes

Overcoming Anxiety, Stress and Panic
A Five Areas Approach

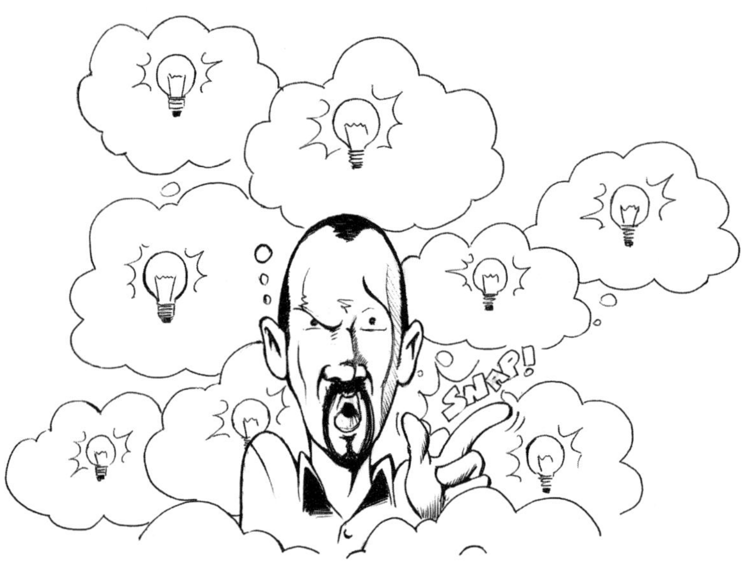

How to start fixing problems and finding solutions (practical problem solving)

www.livinglifetothefull.com
www.fiveareas.com

Dr Chris Williams

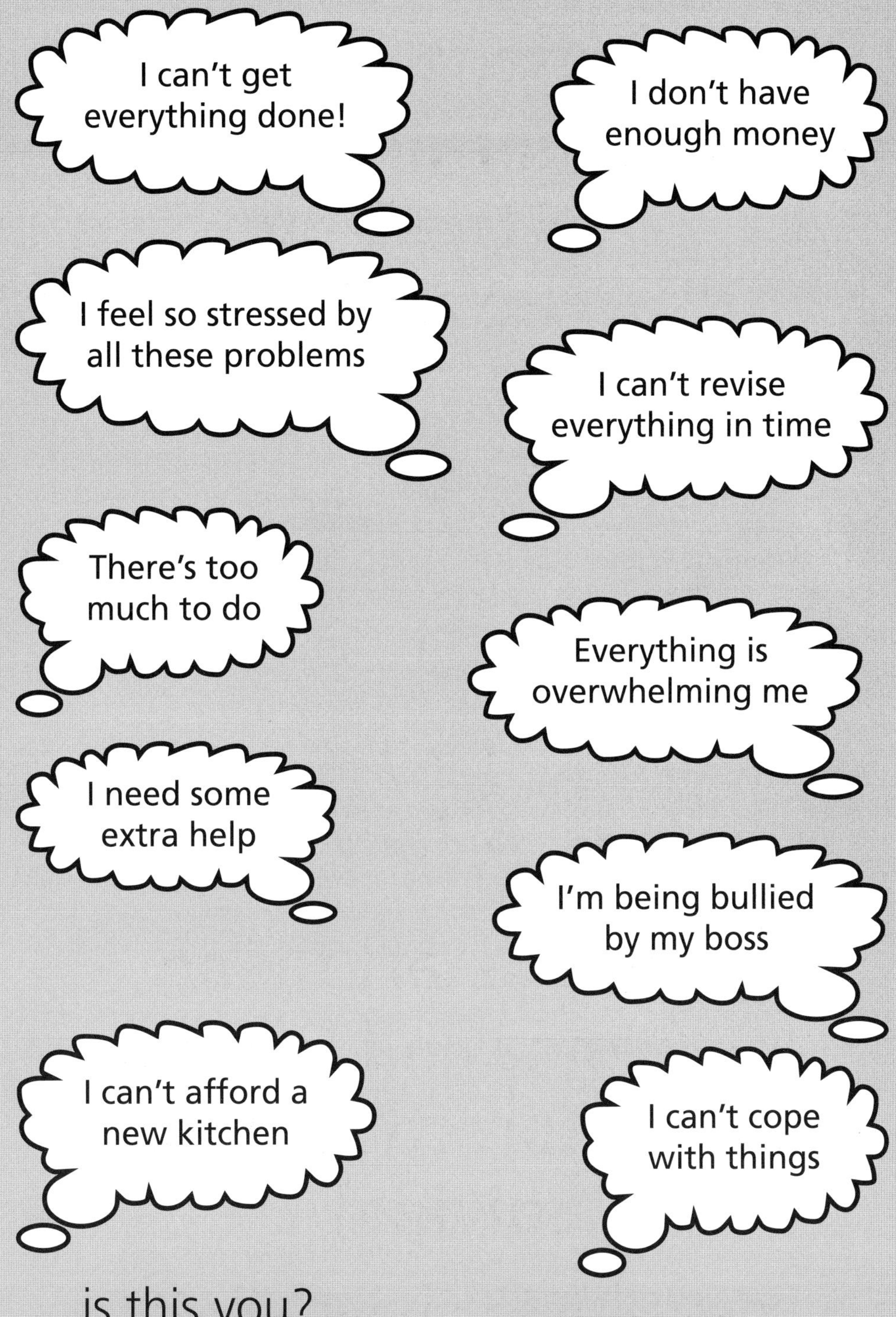
I can't get everything done!
I don't have enough money
I feel so stressed by all these problems
I can't revise everything in time
There's too much to do
Everything is overwhelming me
I need some extra help
I'm being bullied by my boss
I can't afford a new kitchen
I can't cope with things

... is this you?

If so ... this **workbook is for you**.

In this workbook you will:

- Learn how tackling practical problems can help you feel less stressed.
- Learn to recognise problems you can sort out.
- See an example of problem solving in practice and apply it to a problem of your own.
- Learn how to make slow, steady changes to your life.

How problems affect us

Everyone faces some problems in life. It's often easier to cope when there's just one problem. But when you face a particularly hard problem, or a whole lot of smaller ones all at the same time, you can struggle to cope and feel stressed. This is especially so when you are feeling anxious, tired or ground down. Tackling these problems will help you feel better, and this workbook will help you achieve this.

Before you start

Sometimes problems occur because of things you can't control. But sometimes they are the result of things that could have been done differently. For example, problems in relationships may build up because one person kept expecting the other person to do something, but without making it clear what was needed. Perhaps they didn't respond in ways that would have prevented things worsening at an earlier stage. Or maybe a problem of debt has built up because of problem gambling or drinking.

So before you start working towards how to solve your problem, you need to think about these three things:

1. **Your behaviour**: Do you find that the same kinds of problem happen again and again? If so, is there anything that you keep doing (or not doing) that leads to the problem? If you answered 'Yes', you may find the workbook on *Things you do that worsen your anxiety* (*unhelpful behaviours*) useful.
2. **Your thinking**: Is your problem really such an issue? Is it possible that things are being blown up out of all proportion because of how you feel inside at the moment? If you think this may be so, then use the *Noticing and changing anxious thinking* workbook to help you get things back into perspective.

3. **Other people and other ways of support**: Some problems are hard to change by yourself. Is there someone around you who could support you if you feel you can't tackle the problem on your own. You can get outside support if someone close to you can't do it – see the list of useful contacts in the *Understanding worry and stress* (page 24) and *Understanding panic and phobias* workbooks (page 57).

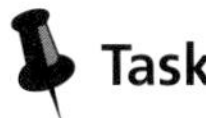

Task

Make a list of any supports and practical resources (for example self-help books) that you have:

Key point

Remember: the supports you have listed may be part of your solution.

How to tackle problems

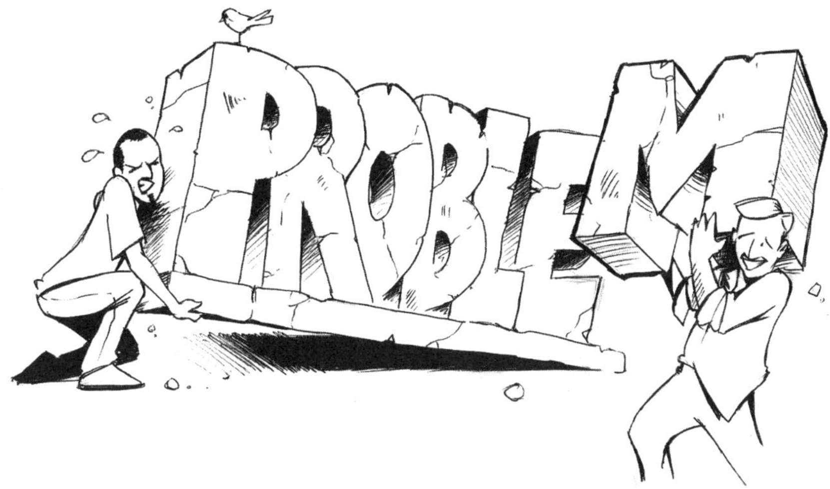

By approaching your practical problems **one step at a time**, you can begin tackling them.

- Approach each problem separately, and in turn.
- Define the problem clearly.
- Break down seemingly enormous and unmanageable problems into smaller parts that are then easier to solve.

Making a plan to tackle problems in a step-by-step way

Setting targets in a planned way can help you decide how to make the changes needed to get better. To do this, set yourself:

- **Short-term** targets – these are changes you can make today, tomorrow and next week.
- **Medium-term** targets – these are changes you could make over the next few weeks.
- **Long-term** targets – this is where you want to be in six months or a year's time.

The seven steps to problem solving

Step 1: Identify and clearly define the problem

Below is a list of common practical and relationship problems that happen when people feel stressed or anxious. Are any of these affecting you? Most people face many issues every day. So it's likely that you will have noticed problems in at least some of these areas.

Practical issues	Yes	No	Sometimes
There's an important task I need to do by a set time	☐	☐	☐
I have worries about money or debts	☐	☐	☐
There are problems where I live	☐	☐	☐
I/somebody close to me doesn't have a job	☐	☐	☐
I/somebody close to me doesn't enjoy their job	☐	☐	☐
I don't have time to do everything needed around the house	☐	☐	☐

Practical issues	Yes	No	Sometimes
I don't have time to do everything needed in my other commitments outside the house/family	☐	☐	☐
There's something I need to buy or borrow	☐	☐	☐
There's too much to do in the available time	☐	☐	☐
There's something practical I don't understand that I need to find out about	☐	☐	☐
There's an item that's broken/damaged/leaking that needs fixing	☐	☐	☐

Relationship issues	Yes	No	Sometimes
There is no-one around who I can really talk to	☐	☐	☐
I have relationship issues (such as arguments) with my partner/spouse	☐	☐	☐
My partner/spouse doesn't really talk to me or offer me enough support	☐	☐	☐
I have relationship issues (such as arguments) with close family members, for example parents/brother/sister	☐	☐	☐
I'm not spending time with my children like I want to	☐	☐	☐
My children won't do what I tell them	☐	☐	☐
Someone close to me has alcohol or drug problems	☐	☐	☐
Someone close to me has problems with the police or courts	☐	☐	☐
Someone close to me is being threatened by somebody	☐	☐	☐
There's someone else (for example a sick relative) I have to care for	☐	☐	☐
I have problems with others, for example neighbours/friends/colleagues at work	☐	☐	☐

Remember, sometimes in anxiety people may avoid or overlook their problems. So go through the list again. Check whether you haven't noted a problem as being a problem because you are avoiding it as a way to cope.

Are there any other practical or relationship problems you need to tackle? Write them down here:

Example: Julia's practical problem

Julia has signed up for a maths course. She wants to try to get an extra qualification to help her get a job she wants to do. She is very anxious about all the revision needed for the exams. She has a busy life that includes looking after her son, Ben, who is 15 years old. She ticks several boxes in the list of problems above, and decides the one she wants to focus on is: **There's an important task I need to do by a set time**. She chooses this problem to tackle first because she has so much to revise before the exams.

Now it's your turn

Look back at your list and choose **one** problem that you will tackle first. This is particularly important if you have ticked many boxes in the list. Trying to overcome all your problems at once can be hard and usually doesn't work. So you need to choose **one** problem to focus on at a time.

My target area: Write down the one problem area you want to work on first.

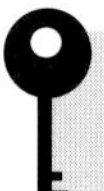

Key point

Choose a practical or relationship problem that is causing you to be distressed now. Write it here:

Well done! By choosing one problem to tackle, you have already started to help reduce your anxiety.

Breaking it down into small steps

Now you need to use a **step-by step** approach to sorting out your problem, where no step seems too large. So you may need to break down your target into many smaller steps that you can tackle one at a time. Remember the first step needs to be something that gets you moving in the right direction.

Example: Julia's step-by-step approach

Julia feels that her problem is too big to sort out in one go. She also knows from reading this course that it's easier to succeed if things are done in a planned way. So she decides to break down the task of revision into smaller steps. As a first step she **writes a revision plan** that will help her get through all the work in time.

Do you need to **break your target into smaller steps**? Answer the following question to help you decide this.

Q Is your problem a clear, focused problem that you can tackle in one go?

Yes ☐ No ☐

If you answered 'Yes', go straight to Step 2. If you answered 'No', think about how you can break the problem into smaller steps. If you need to, write down your new first small step here again:

Step 2: Think up as many solutions as possible to achieve your first target

When you feel overwhelmed by practical problems, often it's hard to see a way out. It can seem hard to even start tackling the problem.

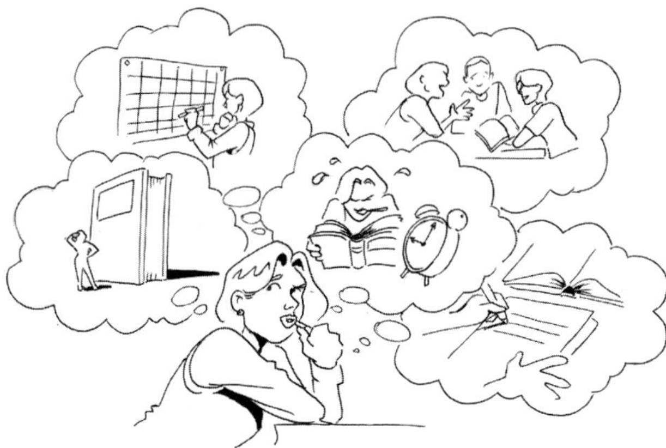

One way around this is to step back from the problem and see what solutions are possible. This is called **brainstorming**. The more solutions that you can think of, the more likely it is that a good one will emerge.

The purpose of brainstorming is to try to come up with **as many ideas as possible**. This makes it easier to identify the solution that should overcome your problem.

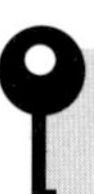

Key point

You can even include ridiculous ideas at first as you are just trying to get yourself to start thinking more flexibly!

Answering the following questions will help you come up with ideas:

- **Q** What advice would you give a friend who was trying to sort out the same problem? Sometimes it's easier to think of solutions for others than for ourselves.
- **Q** What *ridiculous* solutions can you include as well as more sensible ones?
- **Q** What helpful ideas would others (for example, family, friends or colleagues) suggest?
- **Q** What have you tried in the past that was helpful before?

Example: Julia makes a revision timetable – possible solutions

(Including ridiculous ideas at first)

- I could choose to learn absolutely everything from the biggest textbook.
- I could check out the curriculum to help me write a clear plan to revise from.
- I could plan to cram the most important bits into the last few days – and hope I get lucky.
- I could join a revision group of other students and learn with them.
- I could use my lecture notes to decide what topics I want to revise.

Now write down as many possible solutions (including ridiculous ideas at first) for your own problem:

Step 3: Look at the pros and cons of each possible solution

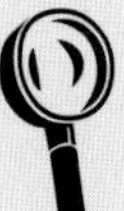

Example: Julia writes down the pros and cons of her solutions

Suggestion	Pros (advantages)	Cons (disadvantages)
I could choose to learn absolutely everything from the biggest textbook	Easier in the short term as I don't have to think much about what to have on the timetable – it's everything!	Well, it would mean revising all the time. This would be stressful. It's a big book and I could never learn it all. And there would be no time for Ben or the flat – or me!
I could check out the curriculum to help me write a clear plan to revise from	This would help me make a clear list of all the topics to cover	I'd need to decide which topics I need to work on and which ones to leave out – some areas are less important
I could plan to cram the most important bits into the last few days – and hope I get lucky	That might work...	That's not a plan, it's a gamble. I'd feel so stressed that I'd be snappy and feel awful
I could join a revision group of other students and learn with them	That's a good idea – I'd get into a routine of working – and we could motivate and test each other	I've got to look after Ben and the flat. So my main chances to revise are later in the evenings. I don't think the groups would be meeting then
I could use my lecture notes to decide what topics I want to revise	That might be a good idea. The lectures did focus on all the key topics on the course.	I missed some of the lectures when Ben was off school ill – but I have most of them

Now write **your own** list of ideas below, and the pros and cons of each suggestion.

My suggestions from Step 2	Pros (advantages)	Cons (disadvantages)

By doing this, you have made a big effort in sorting out your problem.

Step 4: Choose one solution

The best way of tackling a problem is to plan **steady, slow changes**.

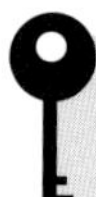

Key point

The solution you are looking for is something that gets you moving in the right direction. This should be small enough to be possible, but big enough to move you forwards. Remember, the purpose of this is to tackle practical problems which are causing you stress and getting you down. Tackle them and you will feel better.

Example: Julia's final choice

Julia tries to choose an option that will make a sensible first step in achieving her goal. She knows her chosen solution should be realistic – only then will it be likely to succeed. She makes her decision after looking at all the pros and cons she's listed in Step 3.

Julia decides to **use her lecture notes to decide what topics to focus on**. Some of the other suggestions might also work, but this suggestion seems the best choice for her.

Look at your own responses in Step 3 and then choose a solution. Write down your own preferred option here:

Now see if you can answer 'Yes' to the first three **Questions for effective change** below.

Will it be *useful* for changing how you are?

Yes ☐ No ☐

Is it a *clear* task so that you will know when you have done it?

Yes ☐ No ☐

Is it something that is realistic, practical and achievable?

Yes ☐ No ☐

If you answered 'Yes' to all three questions, your chosen step should help start you off. If you answered 'No', then think again and choose another option from your list.

Step 5: Plan the steps needed to carry out your chosen solution

You need to have a clear plan that lays out exactly **what** you are going to do and **when** you are going to do it. And an important part of your plan is to predict what would block the plan.

So *write down* the steps needed to carry out your plan. This will help you to:

- Think what to do.
- Predict possible problems that might arise.

That way you can think about how you will respond if there were problems to keep your plan on track.

Example: Julia's plan

Julia gets out her course timetable and looks through the lecture titles. She writes the main topics down on a piece of paper. She then uses the information given to her in the revision lectures to identify the topics the examiners hinted may come up in the exam. She then counts the weeks before the exam – she has eight weeks.

Julia writes down a plan to cover all the key topics over the next seven weeks – this will give her an entire week at the end to revise things again. In each week she works out a realistic amount of time she needs each day to cover each topic – and makes sure she can get through all the main topics in time. She builds in time to learn and also time to test

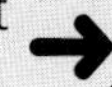

herself. She tries to be realistic in thinking about how much time she will need. Her plan means she will be working between 9pm and midnight every weekday plus half of Saturday each week.

Julia then asks herself if this is a plan that makes clear *what* she is going to do and *when* she is going to do it. She thinks it is.

Julia then asks herself if the plan might be blocked or prevented by anything. She acknowledges that by 9pm she will be quite tired. On balance, she is asking too much of herself. So she goes back to her plan and decides that first, if she falls behind for any reason, she will cut back on two of the less important topics. Second, to avoid getting overly tired, she will ask her mother if Ben can go round to her house three times a week. Then she can work in the early evening rather than later at night. Finally, she builds in some early nights and an evening completely without work in the week – plus Sunday will be off!

Julia looks at her plan again. She feels much better about it and decides to start applying it that evening.

Now, write down your plan here:

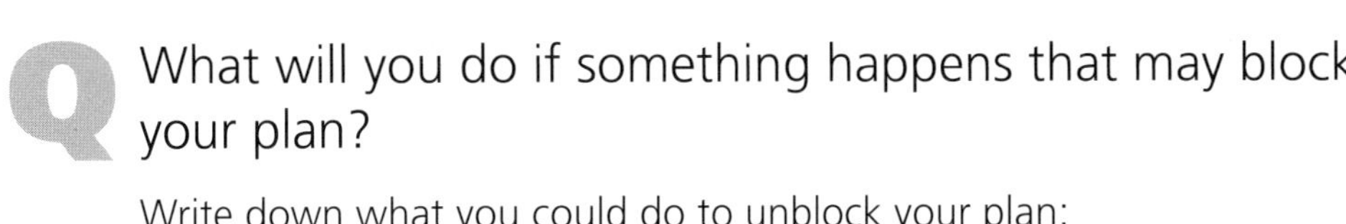

What will you do if something happens that may block your plan?

Write down what you could do to unblock your plan:

Now check your plan against the rest of the **Questions for effective change**.

Is your plan one that:

- Makes clear what you are going to do and when you are going to do it?

  Yes ☐ No ☐

- Won't be easily blocked or prevented?

  Yes ☐ No ☐

- Will help you to learn useful things even if it doesn't work out perfectly?

  Yes ☐ No ☐

If you answered 'Yes' to all three questions, go on to Step 6. If you answered 'No', then think again and try to alter your plan so you answer 'Yes' to all the questions. Remember, you know your life and your plan has to fit around it.

Step 6: Carry out your plan

Now carry out your plan during the next week.

Good luck!

Step 7: Review the outcome

Example: Julia's plan works

Julia starts revising the first topic that evening. Things go really well for the first two weeks. But then Ben is ill and off school for three days. Julia starts to panic about her missed revision work. But she then remembers that she had thought about what she would do if her plan got blocked! So she reviews her timetable. She cuts back on one of the less important topics and starts revising again – keeping to her plan.

By the end of the seventh week Julia has covered everything she had wanted to. This means she hasn't needed to feel too anxious or tired at any stage. She has also really enjoyed the evenings off and has got into the habit of watching a DVD with a friend.

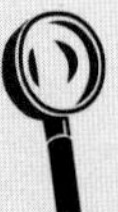

Example 2: Julia's plan doesn't work

Julia starts to carry out her plan. But three weeks into the plan, Ben is involved in a road traffic accident and is seriously ill in hospital. So Julia can't keep to her revision plan. Fortunately, Ben gets better in a few days but will remain in hospital for another 10 days while he recovers from an operation.

Julia thinks "What can I do?". She goes to see her course tutor, who tells her to send in a formal letter explaining her problem along with a letter from the hospital confirming what has happened. She does this and is given the choice of sitting the exam next term. She agrees to this and passes her exam next time.

Now write down your review here:

Q Was your plan successful?

Yes ☐ No ☐

- Did it help improve things?

Yes ☐ No ☐

- Did any problems arise?

Yes ☐ No ☐

What have you learned from doing this?

Write down any helpful lessons or information you have learned. If things didn't go quite as you hoped, try to learn from what happened.

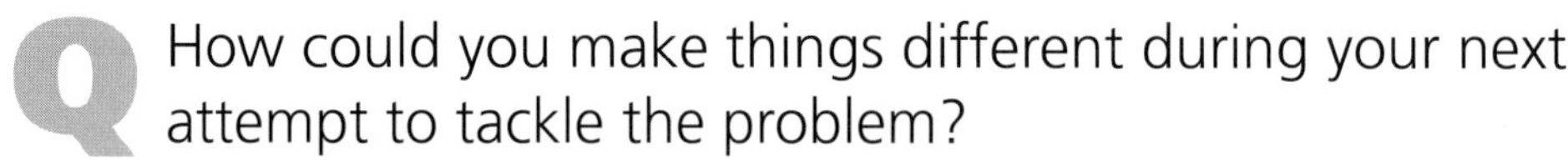

How could you make things different during your next attempt to tackle the problem?

Were you too ambitious or unrealistic in choosing the target you did?

If you noticed problems with your plan

Choosing realistic targets for change is important. This is because if they are realistic, you won't have to worry about them. Think back to where you started – were you too ambitious or unrealistic in choosing the target you did? Sometimes your attempt to solve a problem may be blocked by something unexpected. Perhaps something didn't happen as you planned, or someone reacted in an unexpected way? Try to learn from what happened.

How could you change how you approach the problem to help you make a realistic action plan?

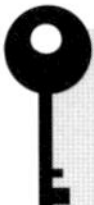

Key point

Remember, most problems can usually be solved – if not in one way then in another.

Planning the next steps

After successfully completing the first round of seven steps, depending on what you have done, you need to plan another change. You will need to slowly build on what you have done in a step-by-step way.

Did your plan help you to tackle the problem you were working on completely? If not, you may need to plan out other solutions to tackle what is left of your problem. The important thing is to **build one step on another**.

So, you now have the choice to:

- Focus on the same problem and plan to keep working on it one step at a time.
- Choose another problem to work on.

Without a step-by-step approach you may find that although you take some steps forward, these can be all in different directions. So to keep your focus and motivation, the steps you decide to take should always be realistic, practical and achievable. Use what you have just learned to build on what you did.

Example: Julia's next steps

Julia's revision plan is now going well.

So she now decides which of her other current problems she will focus on next. She needs to plan to keep up with looking after the flat, which she hasn't been doing while she was focusing on revising for the exam.

Julia creates a new seven-step plan. This includes asking Ben to do more around the flat in return for some trainers she has promised him after she has done the exam. She also says to herself that she won't get upset about it not looking so good – she can always do the essentials and then catch up slowly after the exams are over.

So three months after she made her first plan, Julia is delighted to pass the exam. The flat is also in reasonably good order. Ben is thrilled with his new trainers.

Julia has now sorted out her problem – now it's your turn.

When making your next plan, remember to think of making slow, steady changes. By taking one step at a time, any problem can be dealt with.

Do:

- Plan to work on **only** one or two key problems over the next week. Breaking things down into chunks is a really good way that doesn't add to your anxiety.
- Plan to alter things slowly in a step-by-step way.
- Use the **Questions for effective change** to check that the next step is always well planned.
- Write down your plan in detail so that you know exactly what you are going to do this week.

Don't:

- Try to start to change too many things all at once.
- Choose something that is too hard a target to start with. That will only add to your anxiety.
- Be negative and think 'It's a waste of time'. Try to find out if this negative thinking is actually true.

Write your own short, medium and long-term plans here:

- **Short term** – what might you do over the next week or so? This is your next step that you need to plan.

- **Medium term** – what might you aim towards doing over the next few weeks – the next few steps?

- **Longer term** – where do you want to be in a few months or so?

When you need more help

Remember, you are not alone. If you need more help consider asking:

- People around you, who you know and trust.
- Your GP, health visitor or social worker.

A longer list of supports is provided at the end of the workbooks *Understanding worry and stress* (page 24) and *Understanding panic and phobias* (page 57).

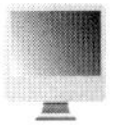

The book *How to Fix Almost Everything* offers even more hints and tips for dealing with practical problems, and includes lots of worked examples. This book and linked free downloadable colour worksheets to help you tackle problems are available from **www.fiveareas.com**.

Credit card-sized versions of the seven steps of problem solving are available for you to print for free or order from the Five Areas website (**www.fiveareas.com**).

Summary

In this workbook you have:

- Learnt how practical problems can worsen anxiety.
- Learnt how to identify problems in your own life that you can change.
- Seen an example of problem solving in practice and applied this to one of your own problems.
- Learnt how to make slow, steady changes to your life.

Q What have I learnt from this workbook?

Q What do I want to try next?

Putting what you have learnt into practice

Continue to put into practice what you learn over the next few weeks. Don't try to solve every problem all at once. Plan out what to do at a pace that's right for you. Build changes one step at a time.

Use the blank summary sheet at the end of the workbook to help you plan your changes. If you are stuck or unsure what to do discuss this with someone else. You can download more sheets for free from **www.fiveareas.com**.

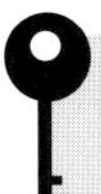

Key point

Don't put off asking for help if you are stuck.

By reading this workbook and following the seven steps approach, you are well on your way to reducing your anxiety, worries or stress.

My notes

The seven steps to practical problem solving worksheet

By working through the seven steps in this worksheet you will learn an approach that will help you to solve your problems. You will need a few sheets of paper and a pen to work through the steps below.

Step 1: Identify and clearly define the problem

- Select the problem area you will tackle.
- Write it down on a separate sheet of paper (page 1).

Do you need to break it down into a smaller target – that is more practical, realistic and achievable in the next week or so? If yes, write down your new target on a new sheet of paper (page 2).

Step 2: Think up as many solutions as possible to achieve your first goal

For this step you will need to **brainstorm** (see page 100 of the workbook). Write down all your solutions as you think of them on a sheet of paper (page 3).

Step 3: Look at the pros and cons of each possible solution

Write down a list of the pros and cons of each option on another sheet of paper (page 4). You can draw a table like the one on page **103** of the workbook.

Step 4: Now choose one of the solutions

Use your answers from Step 3 to make this choice. Write this down on a sheet of paper (page 5) under the heading 'My solution'.

Step 5: Plan the steps needed to carry out your chosen solution

Now on the same page you used in Step 4 (page 5), write down the steps you need to take. Then apply the **Questions for effective change** and write your answers (Yes or No) on the same page.

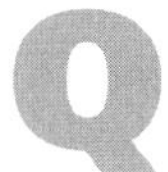

Is your planned activity one that:

- Will be useful for understanding or changing how you are?
- Is a specific task so that you will know when you have done it?
- Is realistic, practical and achievable?
- Makes clear *what* you are going to do and *when* you are going to do it?
- Is an activity that won't be easily blocked or prevented by practical problems?
- Will help you to learn useful things even if it doesn't work out perfectly?

On a new page (page 6) add to the plan that you have written on page 5, a back-up plan of what you will do if your solution **doesn't fully work out**.

Step 6: Carry out your plan

Good luck!

Step 7: Review the outcome

Write down the answers to all the questions below on a sheet of paper (page 7).

- Was the selected solution successful?
- Were there any problems?
- What have you learned from the situation?

Even if the plan wasn't completely successful, there will be things you will have learnt. How can you put what you have learned into practice?

Overcoming Anxiety, Stress and Panic

A Five Areas Approach

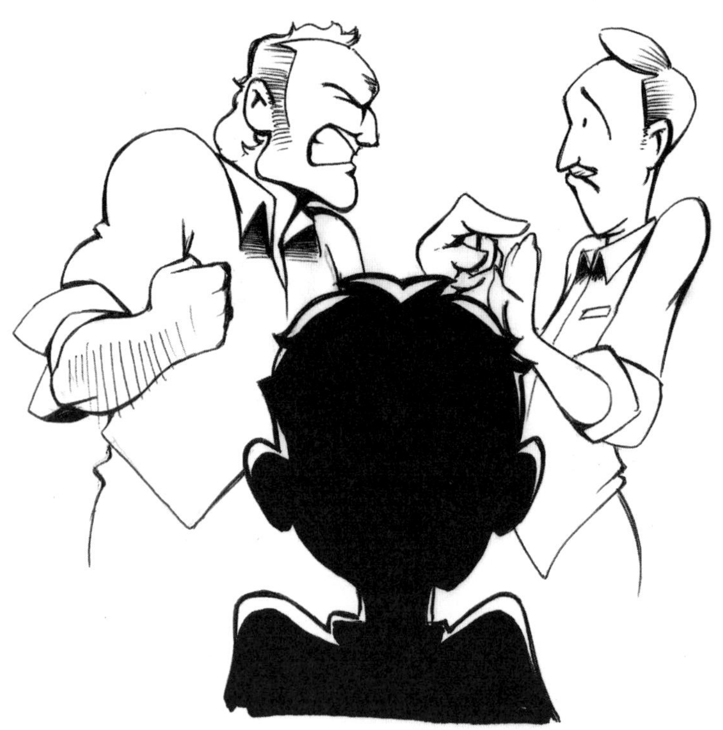

How to ask for what you really need (being assertive)

www.livinglifetothefull.com
www.fiveareas.com

Dr Chris Williams

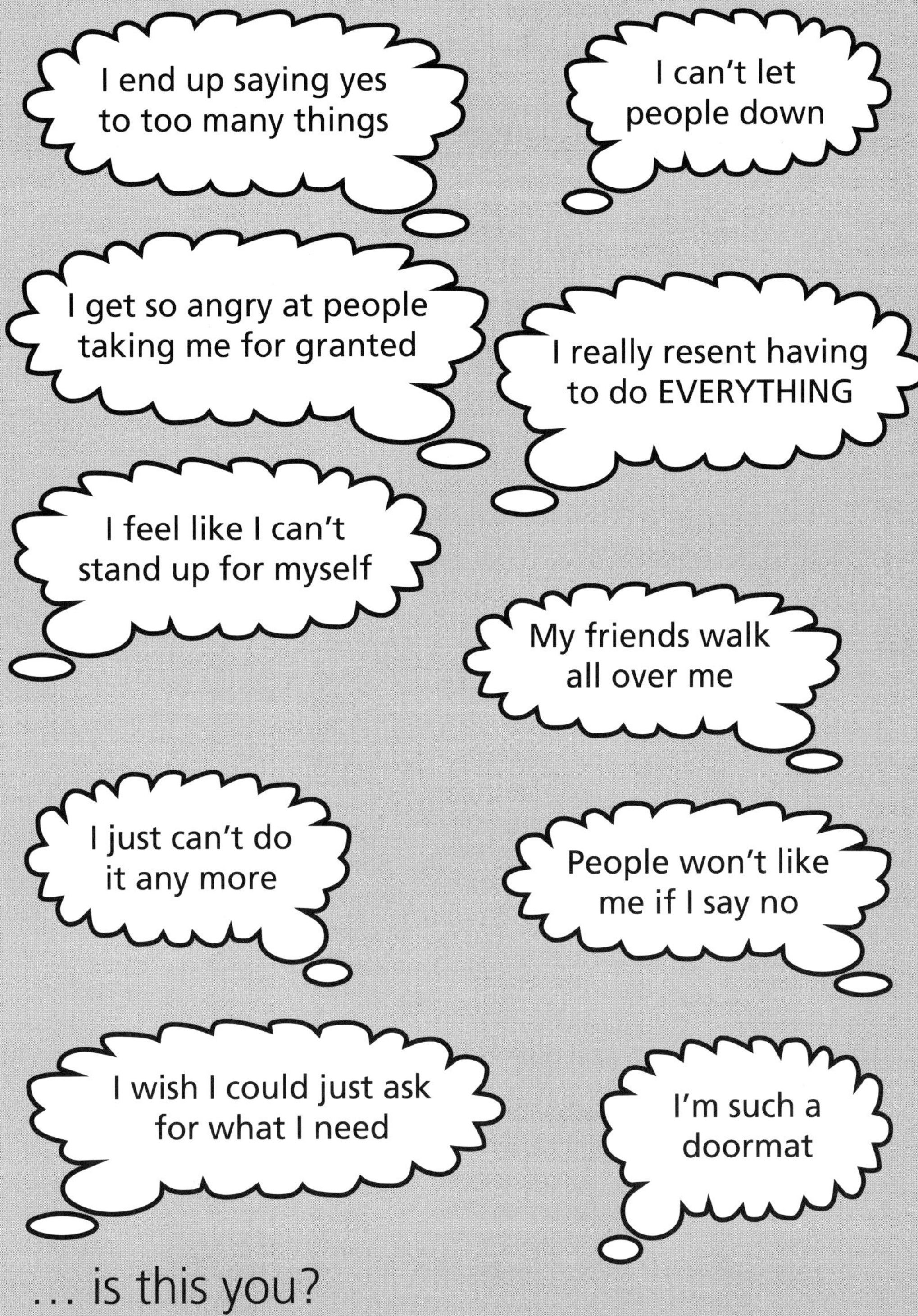
I end up saying yes to too many things
I can't let people down
I get so angry at people taking me for granted
I really resent having to do EVERYTHING
I feel like I can't stand up for myself
My friends walk all over me
I just can't do it any more
People won't like me if I say no
I wish I could just ask for what I need
I'm such a doormat

… is this you?

If so … this **workbook is for you**.

In this workbook you will:

- Learn about the differences between passive and assertive behaviour.
- Learn the rules of assertion and how you can put them into practice in everyday situations.

What is assertiveness?

Assertiveness is being able to:

- Respect yourself and others.
- Stand up for yourself and say what you need clearly.
- Make sure your opinions and feelings are considered.
- Respect others rather than demanding you get what you want.

Key point

You can be assertive without being forceful or rude.

So assertiveness means stating clearly what you need and making sure that what you need is considered **as well as** what other people need.

You can **learn to be and practise being** assertive. By practising being assertive, you'll become more aware of your own needs as an individual.

What do you do in difficult situations?

However confident you are, there are certain situations which many people find it hard to deal with. For example:

- Dealing with unhelpful shop assistants.
- Planning to have *you* time away from your family.
- Asking for help when you need it.
- Asking someone to return something they have borrowed.

- Letting your family or friends know how you feel and what you need.
- Saying no to other people's demands.

Do you often deal with these situations by saying nothing or by **giving in**? If you do, have you noticed that it can leave you feeling unhappy, resentful or out of control? You can feel upset, and then upset other people. Also, avoiding an issue by saying 'Yes' when you mean 'No' often actually doesn't solve your problem.

Sometimes instead of bending over backwards to please people, you may find that time and time again you get angry at people. You may be irritable, rude or complain all the time. If you tend to do this, you will find the workbook *Learning to be calmer, less annoyed and less irritated* helpful.

How can you become more assertive?

While growing up, people learn to relate to others from their family, teachers and friends. You may also be influenced by other things such as TV and magazines. You may have read about how important it is to act or look a particular way and do a great job all the time. But in trying to do this, you can become so focused on doing things for other people that you may forget to do things for yourself as well.

Sometimes your confidence can get worn away. For example if someone has been bullied or ridiculed when they were growing up, or is criticised a lot by their family. You can end up worrying that others won't like you or want to know you unless you are nice to them all the time. You come to believe that if you ever say no then people will get angry, hurt or walk away. This anxiety comes to dominate how you relate to others and you end up feeling like a doormat – always needing to please others – rather than doing what you want.

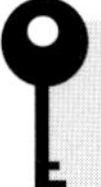

Key point

The good news is that although you may have learned to say 'Yes' when you mean 'No', you can become more assertive by learning **assertiveness skills**.

Key elements of passive behaviour

Behaving passively means:

- Always saying 'Yes'.
- Not letting others know about your feelings, needs and opinions.
- Always choosing others' needs over your own.

Usually people behave passively to **avoid conflict** at all times and to **please others**. You feel anxious and unconfident in your relationships and friendships with others. This kind of behaviour is driven by a fear of not wanting to upset others or have others not like you. But in the longer term, it can make you feel worse.

When someone behaves passively it can cause others to become irritated and have a lack of respect for the person behaving passively. When you behave passively, others can take you for granted and increasingly expect you to drop everything to help them.

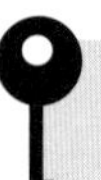

Key point

Being passive can be changed by learning the skill of 'assertive communication'.

Key elements of assertive behaviour

Assertiveness means:

- Letting others know about your feelings, needs and opinions while maintaining respect for other people.
- Expressing your feelings in a direct, honest and appropriate way.
- Realising it's possible to stand up for your opinions in such a way that you don't disregard another person's view at the same time.

Assertion is **not about winning**, but is about being able to walk away feeling that you put across what you wanted to say.

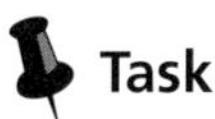

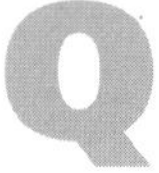

Try to think about a time when someone else has been assertive with you and respected your opinion. How did you feel about them and yourself?

About me – I felt:

About them – I felt:

Benefits of being assertive

Assertiveness is an **attitude** towards yourself and others that is helpful and honest. When you are being assertive, you ask for what you want:

- Directly and openly.
- Appropriately, respecting everyone's opinions and rights, and expecting others to do the same.
- Confidently, without undue anxiety.

By being assertive, you try not to:

- Disregard other people's rights.
- Expect other people to magically know what you want.
- Freeze with anxiety and avoid problems.

Being assertive improves your self-confidence and others' respect for you.

The rules of assertion

The following 12 rules can help you live your life more assertively.

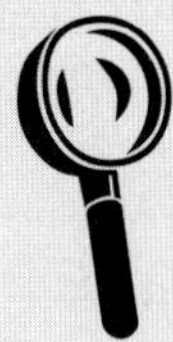

I can:

- Respect myself – who I am and what I do.
- Recognise my own needs as an individual, that is, separate from what's expected of me in particular roles, such as 'mother', 'brother', 'partner', 'daughter', 'son'.
- Make clear 'I' statements about how I feel and what I think, for example 'I feel very uncomfortable with your decision'.
- Allow myself to make mistakes, recognising that it's normal to make mistakes.
- Change my mind, if I choose.
- Ask for 'thinking about it time'. For example, when people ask you to do something, you have the right to say 'I would like to think it over and I will let you know by the end of the week'.
- Allow myself to enjoy my successes, that is, being pleased with what I've done and sharing it with others.
- Ask for what I want, rather than hoping someone will notice what I want.
- Recognise that I am not responsible for the behaviour of other adults or for pleasing other adults all the time.
- Respect other people and their right to be assertive and expect the same in return.
- Say I don't understand.
- Deal with others without depending on them for approval.

At the moment, how much do you believe in each of these rules, and do you put them into practice?

I can:	Do I believe this rule is true?		Have I applied this in the last week?	
Respect myself	Yes ☐	No ☐	Yes ☐	No ☐
Recognise my own needs as an individual independent of others	Yes ☐	No ☐	Yes ☐	No ☐
Make clear 'I' statements about how I feel and what I think, for example 'I feel very uncomfortable with your decision'	Yes ☐	No ☐	Yes ☐	No ☐
Allow myself to make mistakes	Yes ☐	No ☐	Yes ☐	No ☐
Change my mind	Yes ☐	No ☐	Yes ☐	No ☐
Ask for 'thinking about it time'	Yes ☐	No ☐	Yes ☐	No ☐
Allow myself to enjoy my successes	Yes ☐	No ☐	Yes ☐	No ☐
Ask for what I want, rather than hoping someone will notice what I want	Yes ☐	No ☐	Yes ☐	No ☐
Recognise that I am not responsible for the behaviour of others or for pleasing others all the time	Yes ☐	No☐	Yes ☐	No ☐
Respect other people and their right to be assertive and expect the same in return	Yes ☐	No ☐	Yes ☐	No ☐
Say I don't understand	Yes ☐	No ☐	Yes ☐	No ☐
Deal with others without depending on them for approval	Yes ☐	No ☐	Yes ☐	No ☐

You can put these rights into practice to develop assertiveness skills by using assertiveness techniques. Some of these are described below. But before learning the techniques, it's important to know how to start a conversation.

Meeting new people and starting conversations

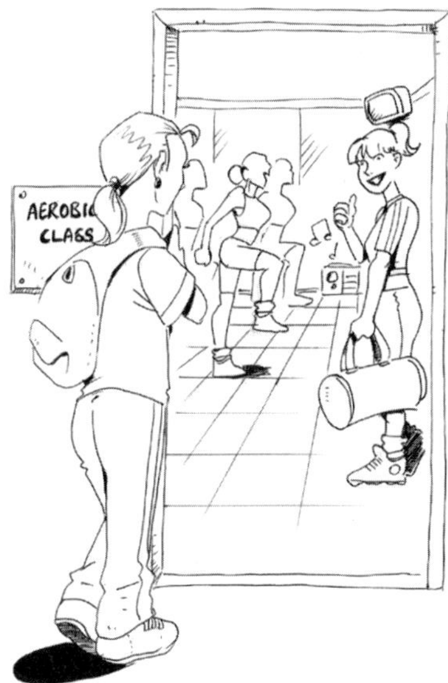

Sometimes you can feel isolated if there is no-one around to talk to. You may feel lonely but you lack contact with anyone. There are many practical things you can do to begin to meet people. For example:

- Making friends through people you know already.
- Joining an aerobics class or some other group sport at your local leisure centre or a playgroup if you have small children.
- Doing a course, such as an adult evening class to learn a new language or joining a club, for example at your local community hall.
- Visiting other local places where you can meet people, for example community organisations or the local place of worship. Some local shops such as post offices, pharmacies and hairdressers also provide a place to talk.
- Think about where you sit when you go to these classes, courses, places or events. It's going to be hard to chat to anyone if you sit by yourself. Make a choice to move closer, and to ask – and answer – questions.
- Getting in touch with people you know but haven't seen for a while. Use email, write a letter or telephone to get in touch. Arrange to meet if you can.
- Don't rush it – but remember confidence comes with doing. It takes time to get to know people and develop friendships.

Here are some good conversation starters:

- How are you?
- Nice day, isn't it?
- Hi, I'm new here and a little bit nervous.
- How old is your baby? He looks so alert.

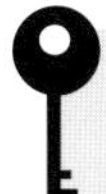

Key point

Remember – it doesn't matter if you talk about superficial things to begin with, such as the weather, the local news or about a holiday. The key is breaking the ice. Also don't worry if there's a pause in the conversation. It's quite okay to just 'be'.

You can also think of some **conversation starters in advance**. Good opening questions often begin with the words:

- **What?** – what was the meeting like last week? What did you do yesterday? What was the new film like?
- **How?** – how did you find the meal? How are you? How are you getting on with the decorating?
- **When?** – when will we be covering this on the course? When do you start back at work?
- **Who?** – who came yesterday? Who's that over there?
- **Why?** – why does that happen (or not happen)? Why do we do things this way?

Then follow these with **back-up questions**. For example:

- Who came yesterday – did they enjoy it?
- What did they say?
- Did it go well?
- Do you think they'll come back?

Practise getting into conversations before going on to the next part of this workbook.

Assertiveness techniques you could use

Now that you have learned to get into conversation you can start to practise being assertive – well done! The following assertiveness techniques will help you to build assertive communication into what you say.

'Broken record'

First, practise what you want to say by repeating over and over again what you want or need. During the conversation, keep returning to your prepared lines, stating clearly what it is you need or want. Do not be put off by clever arguments or by what the other person says. Once you have prepared the lines you want to say, you can relax. This works in virtually any situation.

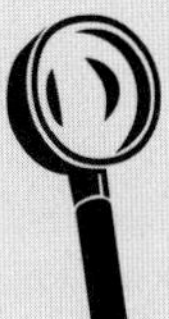

Example: Being firm about what you want

Raj: 'Can I borrow £10 from you?'

Paul: 'I cannot lend you any money. I've run out.'

Raj: 'I'll pay you back as soon as I can. I need it desperately. You are my friend aren't you?'

Paul: 'I cannot lend you any money.'

Raj: 'I would do the same for you. You won't miss £10.'

Paul: 'I am your friend but I cannot lend you any money. I'm afraid I've run out.'

Remember

- Work out beforehand what you want to say.
- Repeat your reply over and over again and stick to what you have decided to say.

Saying 'No'

Many people find that 'No' seems to be one of the hardest words to say. Try to remember when you may have found yourself in situations that you didn't want to be in, just because you had avoided saying this one simple word.

Why does this happen? People often worry that they may be seen as being mean and selfish, or they may worry about being rejected by others. They may notice feelings of false guilt and feel bad that they are letting people down. False guilt means that you feel guilty when you haven't actually done anything wrong. False guilt and anxiety can lead you to apologise when you don't need to, and say 'Yes' to things you don't really want to do.

Key point

Saying 'no' can be both important and helpful. It can protect you from people who will take advantage of you, and help you focus on the important commitments you really want to do.

Task

Q Do I have problems saying 'No'?

Yes ☐ No ☐ Sometimes ☐

If you ticked 'Yes' or 'Sometimes', try to practise saying 'No' by using the following techniques:

- Be straightforward and honest so that you can make your point effectively.
- Your feelings of anxiety may make it seem to you that you are being rude if you say 'No'. Remember that asking for what you need politely and assertively isn't the same as being rude.
- Tell the person if you are finding it hard.
- Don't apologise and give all sorts of reasons for saying 'No'. It is okay to say 'No' if you don't want to do things. Then leave it at that.
- Remember that it is better in the long run to be truthful than breed resentment and bitterness within yourself.

Body language and assertiveness

How people communicate involves more than just words. The tone of your voice, how quickly and loudly you speak, eye contact and body posture – all affect how you come across. When you're being assertive be aware of the non-verbal communications you make as well as the words you say.

Eye contact

- Meet the other person's eyes from time to time.
- Make eye contact – but don't end up staring at the person.
- Try not to look down for long – this may seem rude to others.

If you find this hard to do, practise looking just past the person. For example, look at a thing such as a picture on the wall behind them. This shows you are paying attention – but without directly meeting the other person's eyes.

Your voice

- Try to vary your tone so you come over as interested and interesting.
- Don't be afraid of silence – especially if you've asked a question. When you ask a question you may be tempted to fill any uncomfortable gaps yourself. Be prepared to allow a little silence. Likewise, you don't need to reply instantly to any question. Remember that you're allowed some time to think.
- Think about how quickly or loudly you talk. Aim for a relaxed yet serious manner if you can.

Posture

Think about how you hold your body:

- Try looking up and don't hunch over – this can happen when you feel vulnerable or anxious.
- Keep an appropriate distance ('personal space') between you and the other person.
- Don't get too close – this might be seen as aggressive or inappropriate (unless you know the person very well).

Be friendly

Smiling once in a while is okay.

Be relaxed in your body

- Think about how you hold your body. If you're tense or anxious you may clench your fists and frown, which may come over as being aggressive.
- Relax your body. Quickly think about how you are holding your arms and shoulders and try to relax tense muscles. Some people tend to pull up their shoulders towards their ears when they feel tense.

A word of caution

Don't think you have to suddenly get all of this right straight away. You should make these changes slowly – over many weeks or even months.

Don't get too worried about whether you are making eye contact enough. All you need to do is be aware of this, and occasionally make some small changes in what you do. Experiment and see what works best for you.

Trying out being more assertive

Think about the following when you plan to respond assertively. Choose:

- **The right person**. Some people can take even assertive feedback badly. If you know that what you say is likely to be misinterpreted or that the person is prone to over-react to things then you need to get some extra help, such as from a close friend or a family member.
- **The right time**. For example, try not to start talking about important things as soon as your partner gets in from work or from an evening out and is feeling tired or has been drinking. Choose a more relaxed time – or plan such a time – for example during a meal or walk together.
- **The right issue**. The issue needs be something that the other person can change. For example, asking your mother to look after your baby at times when she has to go to work is not realistic. Instead, choose a time that will suit you both.
- **The right words**. Use the approaches described in this workbook ('Broken record' and 'Saying No'). These techniques will help you to say what you need.

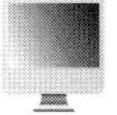

Credit card-sized versions of the rules of assertion and the seven steps of problem solving are available for you to print for free or order from the Five Areas website (**www.fiveareas.com**).

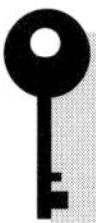

Key point

If you are in a relationship with someone who is violent towards you or others, you may find it impossible to be assertive. This is a situation where you need more help – from social services, the police, your doctor or others. Don't be afraid to ask for help if you can't manage being assertive yourself – it's okay to do so.

Summary

In this workbook you have learnt:

- The differences between passive and assertive behaviour.
- About the rules of assertion and how you can put them into practice in everyday life.

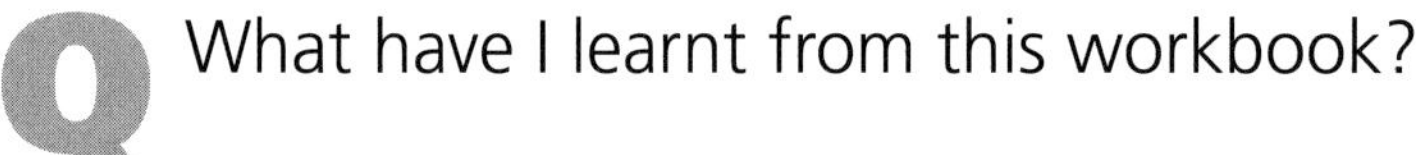

Q What have I learnt from this workbook?

Q What do I want to try next?

Putting into practice what you have learned

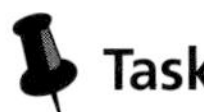

Task

Read again what you learned earlier in the workbook about the 'Broken record' and 'Saying No' approaches, and try to put them into practise during the next week. Think about other ways you can be more assertive in your own life.

If you recognise that you lack assertiveness, try to:

- Use one of the two assertiveness techniques during the next week.
- Remind yourself about and put into practise the *rules of assertion*. Copy page 124 or tear it out and carry it around with you. Put it somewhere you will see it (for example, by your TV or on a door or mirror or on the fridge) to remind you of these rules.

View this as an action plan that can help you to change how you are and also to learn something new about yourself and other people.

My notes

Overcoming Anxiety, Stress and Panic

A Five Areas Approach

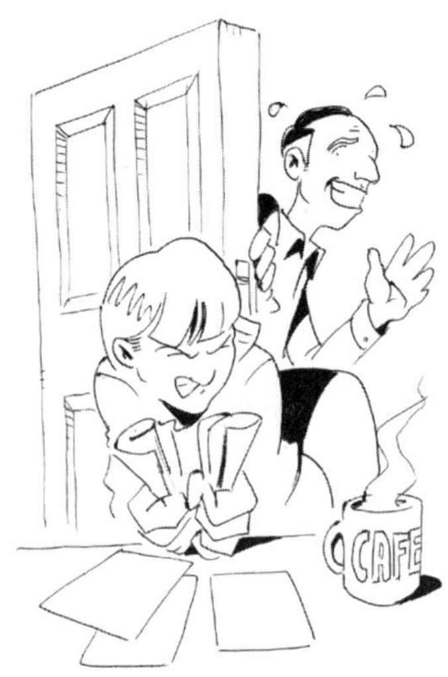

Learning to be calmer, less annoyed and less irritated

www.livinglifetothefull.com
www.fiveareas.com

Dr Chris Williams

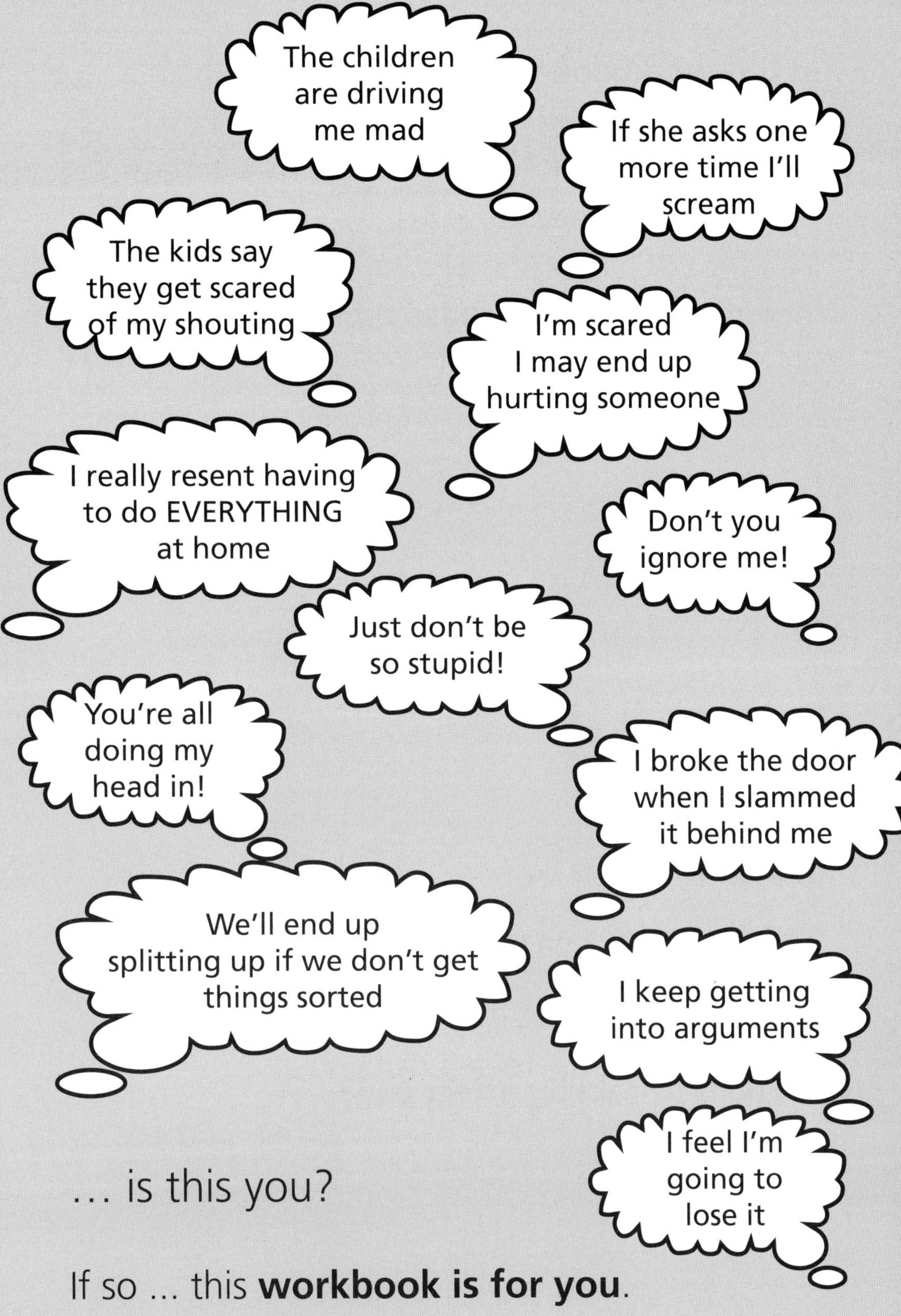
The children are driving me mad
If she asks one more time I'll scream
The kids say they get scared of my shouting
I'm scared I may end up hurting someone
I really resent having to do EVERYTHING at home
Don't you ignore me!
Just don't be so stupid!
You're all doing my head in!
I broke the door when I slammed it behind me
We'll end up splitting up if we don't get things sorted
I keep getting into arguments
I feel I'm going to lose it

... is this you?

If so ... this **workbook is for you**.

In this workbook you will:

- Learn how getting annoyed and irritable can cause you problems.
- Discover situations that make you prone to being irritable or snappy.
- Learn some ways of tackling irritability.

When does irritability cause problems?

Anyone can feel irritable, snappy or annoyed from time to time. But sometimes people or events can make these feelings even worse. For example, there may be just too much to do. Feeling stressed or low can also make you feel more irritable than usual.

If you are more irritable than before, this workbook will help you get back on track. This includes when:

- Smaller and smaller frustrations set you off.
- You become snappy or lash out in words or actions without thinking.
- You feel you are starting to lose control.
- Your irritability is making things worse for you and others around you.

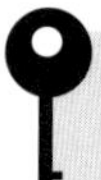

Key point

Sometimes feelings of irritability and anger are linked to serious problems such as being dependent on alcohol or drugs, or to other severe mental health problems. If you are close to hurting yourself or anyone else, it's very important that you discuss with your healthcare practitioner what other supports and treatments can help you.

How does irritability affect you?

Sometimes people can fall into patterns of being snappy and irritable about things. Certain people or events can frustrate you – and you can fall into the trap of responding angrily again and again ... and again. To break a pattern of behaviour, first you need to be aware that it is happening. Two common patterns to watch out for are:

- Depression – which can lead to feeling more irritable, stressed and low, especially first thing in the day.
- Drinking too much, or using street drugs such as amphetamines and cocaine – which can make you feel more irritable. Some prescribed drugs such as steroids can also cause this.

It can be helpful therefore to 'play detective' – try to work out if you feel worse:

- Regularly at any time of day
- When faced by particular people or situations
- Within a couple of hours of using drink, tablets or street drugs.

Spotting patterns of irritability

Use the Irritability diary at the end of the workbook to record **all the times** when you are feeling more irritable or snappy over the next few days. Also record how you deal with these feelings. For example:

- Keeping it to yourself and saying nothing.
- Raising your voice or shouting.
- Saying things in a nasty tone of voice (for example, being sarcastic, cutting, icy or mocking).
- Swearing at yourself or at the situation.
- Swearing or insults aimed directly at someone else.
- Hitting, pushing or throwing an object, or slamming a door (for example, hitting a jammed printer, throwing a book or kicking a ball away).

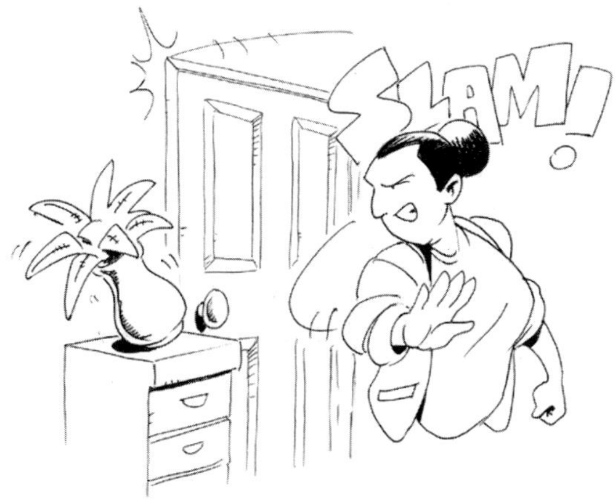

- Deliberately breaking something that belongs to others.
- Making threatening eye contact.
- Moving closer and being physically intimidating.
- Complaining about others to their face.
- Complaining to others under your breath, or behind their back.
- Getting back at someone in an indirect way (for example, refusing help at a later time).
- Doing something to block how frustrated you feel (for example, having a drink).

Try to record **every time** you feel irritated or are snappy. Make a note of what led up to this, and how you reacted. For an example of a completed diary, see Helen's Irritability diary on page 140.

Example: Helen rates her irritation

Helen and Paul have lived together for several years. For the past six months Paul has struggled with illness and has been off work. Helen is irritated that he is around so much at home. She feels Paul interferes with her work as a book-keeper. At the moment she is falling behind on an important job that she has to complete by the end of Tuesday.

Helen's Irritability diary shows that there are certain things that make the irritability worse and which she can therefore plan to change.

Helen feels over-worked and has too much to do. She needs to tell Paul that until Tuesday she has to have lots of planned, uninterrupted time to get on with her work. After Tuesday, she could create a timetable that includes times when she isn't working when she and Paul could talk, go for a walk, etc.

As Helen completes the diary, she realises that the deadline she has set is partly her own fault. She had suggested she could get the accounts for the year back to the client by Tuesday at 5pm. They didn't actually need them by then – but that's when she had promised them. She is pretty sure no-one will actually look at them until the end of the week or even →

later. She feels guilty about the idea of contacting the client to see if she could return them later.

Am I drinking too much caffeine or alcohol, or using street drugs?

Caffeine is a chemical stimulant which is found in tea, coffee, chocolate, as well as hot chocolate and cola drinks. In smaller quantities it makes you feel more alert. However, higher levels can prevent sleep and make your sleep unrefreshing. Higher levels can also lead you to feel more irritable and snappy.

If you drink more than five cups of strong coffee every day for several weeks or months, and then reduce the amount suddenly, you can get caffeine withdrawal. You may feel more irritable, have headaches, not feel like sleeping, sweat a lot and feel fidgety.

Helen has been having more than five cups of strong coffee every day. It is therefore sensible for her to reduce this towards five or fewer cups a day. She should do this slowly by changing over one cup a day to decaffeinated coffee or tea every five or six days. In this way the changes are made slowly but steadily. A change to cold water can also be refreshing. Drinking properly is also good for the body. It boosts alertness and tackles tiredness.

Helen has also noticed that she is drinking alcohol sometimes just to cope. Alcohol can reduce stress in the short term. But it can also make you less restrained (disinhibited). When people are disinhibited, they can say things or make decisions that they later regret. Drinking a lot day in and day out, or using drugs such as cocaine/amphetamines, can also make you more irritable, anxious, tense or depressed. You can find out more about this in the *Stress, alcohol and drugs* workbook.

Is poor sleep and tiredness making me more irritable?

Sleeplessness is a common cause of irritability. A bad night's sleep is a poor start to any day. Helen has noticed that on the second day she felt far less tired in the morning as she had slept better. This helped her not to feel so irritable until later on in the day, when she feels more tired. She can make useful changes to her sleep pattern and the worries that cause her to stay awake using the *How to get a good night's sleep: overcoming anxiety and sleep problems workbook*.

Example: Helen's Irritability diary

Date and time	Record your recent sleep/drink and feelings of pressure leading up to the irritation	People and events leading up to feeling irritable	My feelings at the time	My thoughts at the time	Altered physical symptoms	My altered behaviour
	Are you feeling tired? Have you been drinking alcohol or caffeine? Are you feeling pressured or hassled leading up to the time you felt annoyed?	– Where were you? – Who were you with? – What were you doing? – What was said /happened?	How did you feel emotionally at the time? – Were you irritable, annoyed or angry? – Any other emotions (anxious, ashamed, depressed, or guilty)?	Any thoughts about: – Things not being fair? – Being picked on or mocked? – Being ignored? Or about: – How you are coping? – The worst that could happen? – How others see you? – Your own body, behaviour or performance? – Any memories or mental pictures?	Note down any strong physical symptoms you noticed at the time, e.g. tension, rapid heartbeat, breaking out in a sweat, breathing faster, feeling shaky.	– What did you do differently? – What did you say differently – and how did you say it? – Did you stop doing what you were doing, or start doing something different?

Example: Helen's Irritability diary *continued*

Monday 9am	Poor sleep last night worrying about workload. 1 cup of coffee with breakfast. Half bottle wine last night. Definitely felt hassled – I had too much to do	I was starting work and had booted up the computer in the home office. Lots to do. Paul was hanging about and chatting, stopping me from working	Annoyed and frustrated.	I need to get on. Doesn't he know he's irritating me? Someone has got to bring the money in. It's not fair for him to do this.	Feeling tense and fidgety	Was quite short with Paul and tried to ignore him by looking at the screen and only answering with one word answers. He got the point and left.
Monday 12.00	Even more tired after a morning without a break. three cups of coffee that morning. No alcohol. Felt hassled – just too much to do again	Working in the study. Paul came by and wanted us to go for a walk and lunch at the pub.	Ratty/irritable. Guilty a bit too.	It's all well for him to want me to take time off – he's not working! I've not enough time to do this. It's unfair of him to ask. I've too much to do. He's so selfish.	Feeling tense, hot and breathing faster.	Was snappy and said that I've got too much to do. Suggested he goes out himself if he has so little to do (sarcastically). Paul then got annoyed and said I was being selfish and unsupportive – and stormed out.

Example: Helen's Irritability diary *continued*

Monday 8pm	Another exhausting day. Eight cups of tea and coffee during the day. No alcohol. Still very aware of what hasn't been done and feeling	Paul sits in the chair watching TV and not saying much.	Feel frustrated by his lack of motivation.	He's getting so lazy and letting himself go. He's not applied for a job for a week.	Feel tension in my forehead.	Choose not to act annoyed. Asked him in a friendly voice about his walk Apologised for being ratty and said I'd slept poorly. pressured. He seemed a lot perkier and we had a good chat. I felt stressed and drank a bottle of wine to get me off to sleep.
Tuesday 4.30pm	Feeling very tired. Slept badly last night again worrying about the work. Had 3 cups of coffee today, but no alcohol. Very hassled – trying to beat the 5pm deadline.	Phone call comes from client asking when accounts will be ready. I don't have them quite finished so say I will send them tonight – then get angry at myself for not asking for extra time to do them properly during work time.	Anxious, angry	I've got to get this done. I'll be letting them down if they don't get it when I said I'd send it. I can't do all this. Angry at myself for not getting this sorted sooner. Angry at the client because I didn't ask them for an extension. Angry at Paul for being here.	Tense, sweaty, heart racing, feeling a little sick.	Got distracted, had to start the month again. Ended up missing deadline, and working till 11.30pm. Was so annoyed I hit the table with my hands and felt near to tears.

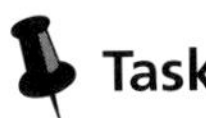

Task

Now keep your own Irritability diary for the next few days. Use the blank diary at the back of this workbook, or copy it. You can download more for free from **www.fiveareas.com**.

How the diary can help you move forwards

Use your diary to discover **patterns** in what you do and don't do.

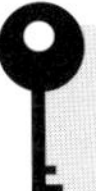

Key point

Keeping a diary can help you find out which activities or situations make you feel more ratty and irritable. If you find you are under pressure and have limited time, then just record key words to help you remember, or fill it in when you are forced to stop, such as when using the toilet or having a bath.

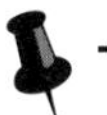

Task

Write down what patterns you discover here:

Do any of your difficult times or situations happen again and again? (For example, do you feel more annoyed when you are hot or when it's crowded? For example, on a bus or in a crowd? Are you frustrated by the same situation or person/people again and again?)

Do you become more irritable at times of high pressure? (For example feeling hassled, crowded, or under time pressure, etc).

Do you feel worse first thing in the day, or regularly feel worse within a couple of hours of using drink, tablets or street drugs?

Do you have any problems with being assertive or communicating with people? (For example, do you need to say No, or ask to rearrange anything differently to take off the pressure?)

Do you need a planned approach to solving any of your problems? (Can you plan a timetable to work efficiently, whilst also having breaks/time for others/other things?)

Are you drinking too much caffeine or alcohol, or using street drugs? (For example, are you drinking more than five cups of coffee a day? Does drink or alcohol affect how you feel?)

Is poor sleep and tiredness making you more irritable? (If Yes, how can you tackle that?)

Making changes

By answering the questions above, you have now made yourself aware of the reasons that are making you irritable. This is an important step in moving forward so well done!

Now use your answers to the questions above to work out what longer-term changes you need to make in your life. The other workbooks in this course can help you plan these key changes.

The following table lists some of the most useful workbooks for planning changes when you feel more irritable than you want to. Choose the ones you want to work on over the next weeks. Try to go through about one workbook a week.

Workbook	Tick those you plan to read
How to start fixing problems and finding solutions (practical problem solving)	☐
How to ask for what you really need (being assertive)	☐
How to get a good night's sleep: overcoming anxiety and sleep problems	☐
Using exercise to overcome stress	☐
Noticing and changing anxious thinking	☐
Stress, alcohol and drugs	☐

You can also plan to respond differently when you start to feel irritable. To do this you need to:

- Identify your warning signs that you are getting annoyed, and

then:

- Change how you react.

Identifying your warning signs that say STOP NOW

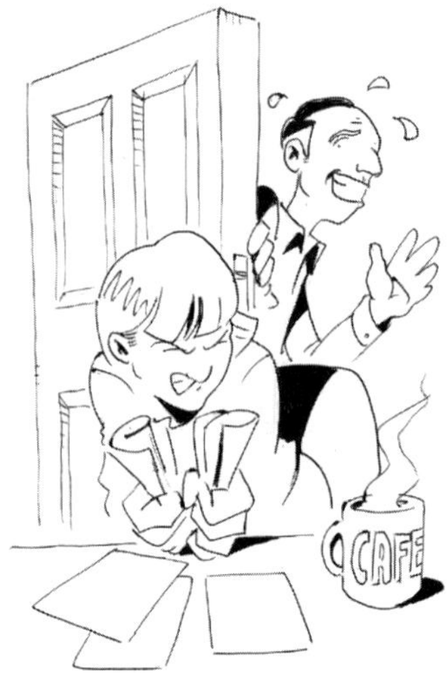

Think back to a recent time when you have felt annoyed. Use your Irritability diary to prompt your memory. Then try to play detective and think about whether there were any 'early warning' signs that you were getting irritable or angry. The key is to try to notice a key reaction or response that you can use as a marker meaning: STOP NOW.

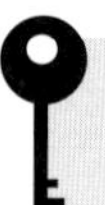

Key point

Early warning signs can include:

- *Altered thinking*: such as thinking something isn't fair, that you are being got at, mocked, humiliated or ignored.
- *Altered emotions/feelings*: of rising irritation, shame, anxiety, panic or anger.
- *Altered physical symptoms*: for example, getting hot, sweaty, fidgety, noticing more rapid breathing or heart rate, or tension.
- *Altered behaviour or activity levels*: for example, pacing, gripping your hands, facing away from the person, drinking more, raising your voice, becoming sarcastic, dismissive or rude.

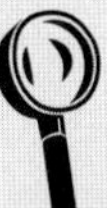

Example: Helen identifies her early warning signs

Helen is working and making good progress. Paul comes in to ask if she wants a coffee. Helen immediately feels hot and flushed and notices a feeling of tension in her forehead. She feels her temper rising but is able to catch herself. She has identified that the tension feeling in her forehead means STOP NOW and do something different instead. Therefore instead of ignoring Paul, and giving one word answers, she forces herself to look away from the computer, smile and say thank you for the offer. He gets her a decaffeinated coffee, and she thanks him and quickly tells him how it is going.

Paul then says he should go because he knows this is a work period for her. He's off to the employment office to attend a course and will be back after lunch. Helen is pleased. She gets a coffee, has a helpful break, and knowing that Paul is away for a time, doing something useful, allows her to keep focused.

Now do some thing different about it

The good news is that you can learn to do something different when you start to feel irritable or angry. The moment you notice your key early warning sign, choose to STOP NOW, like Helen did in the example above. The key is to choose to respond differently. This will help break the pattern that is backfiring on you and those around you.

Here are some suggestions of different responses that can help.

Reduce your body tension

- Drop your shoulders.
- Continue to take normal-sized breaths.
- If you are tensing up, choose to relax your arms or legs.
- In the longer term, learn to use the Anxiety Control Training approach. You can practise this at **www.livinglifetothefull.com** or download free MP3 files from **www.fiveareas.com**. You can also order the 1, 2, 3 Chill audio CD version from there. As you get used to working with the approach you can learn to use the key words 'Calm' and 'Control' to relax very rapidly.

Change the focus of your thoughts

- Choose not to focus on annoyed, hurt or angry thoughts. Say to yourself 'I'm not going down that route again'. Avoid jumping to conclusions and mind-reading. Take a long-term view – it won't matter so much in two weeks. What advice would you give a friend? Apply the same advice to yourself.
- Humming a tune or a favourite song (such as *Jingle Bells*) can help you break out of cycles of upsetting or annoying thinking. This can be helpful to break the cycle of irritation once you have decided on the pointlessness of getting irritated just now.
- Then move your mind onto what else is happening right now, or on doing another activity. You can find more useful hints and tips in the *Noticing and changing anxious thinking* workbook.

Do something different

- If the issue **doesn't really matter** then say 'You're right about that' to the other person. Don't even bother with the argument.
- If the issue really **does matter**, then respond assertively rather than with anger or irritation. Say and ask for what you need. Express your opinion politely and firmly rather than rise to the bait. Don't assume people automatically know what you need.

Assertively expressing what you need and think

Sometimes you can get trapped in old patterns of responding where you quickly feel ratty or irritable. At such times, standing back and thinking about ways of asking for what you need politely and assertively can really help.

Assertiveness is being able to:

- Stand up for yourself.
- Make sure your opinions and feelings are considered.
- Not letting other people always get their way.

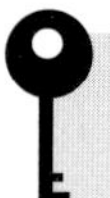

Key point

You can be assertive without being forceful, irritated, angry or rude.

So assertiveness means stating clearly what you expect and making sure that what you want is considered **as well as** what other people want.

You can **learn and practise** being assertive. By practising being assertive, you'll become more aware of your own needs as an individual. You can find out how to become more assertive in the *How to ask for what you really need (being assertive)* workbook.

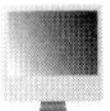

Credit card-sized versions of the rules of assertion and the seven steps of problem solving are available to print for free or order from the Five Areas website (**www.fiveareas.com**).

Summary

In this workbook you have learnt:

- How getting annoyed and irritable can cause you problems.
- About situations that make you prone to becoming irritable or snappy.
- Some ways of tackling irritability.

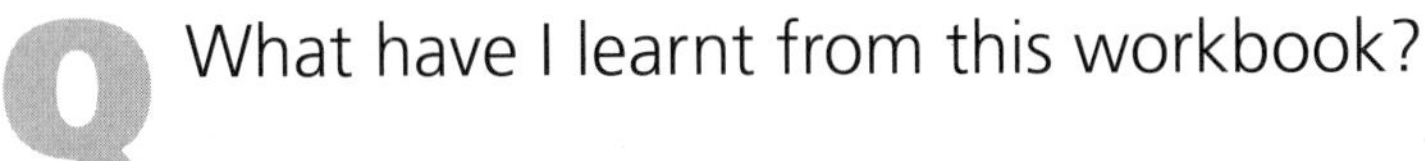

What have I learnt from this workbook?

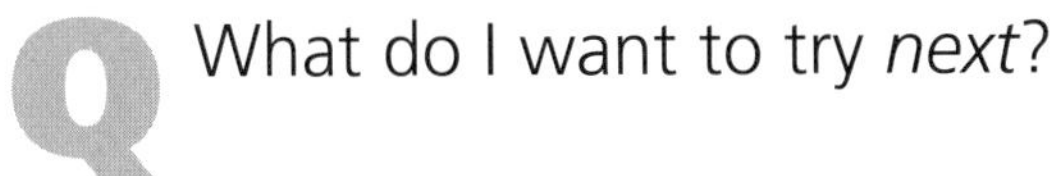

What do I want to try *next*?

Putting what you have learned into practice

Look forward to the **Sleep checklist of things to do and not do** on page 166. Plan to make changes in how you prepare for sleep and what you do once you are in bed.

Write down what you're going to do this week, to put into practice what you have learnt.

My practice plan

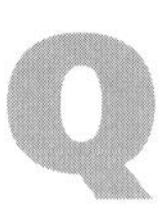

What changes am I going to make?

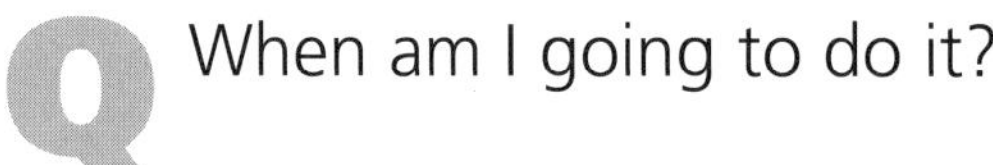

When am I going to do it?

Q What problems could arise, and how can I sort these?

Apply the **Questions for effective change** to your plan.

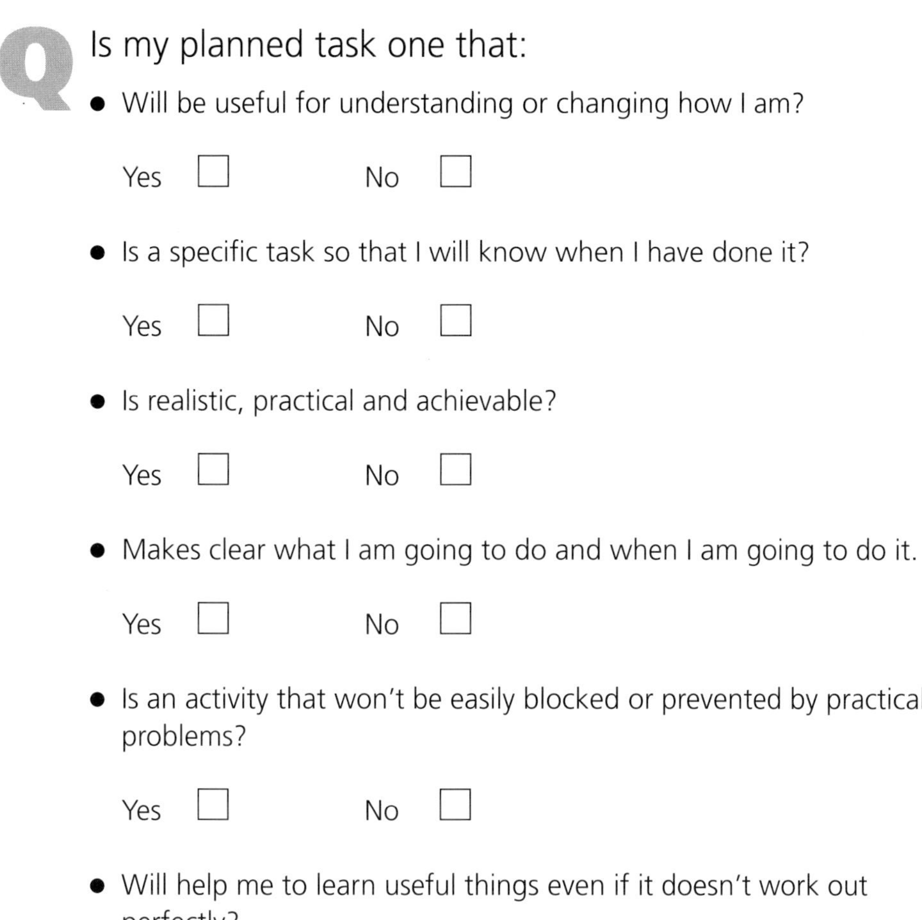

Is my planned task one that:

- Will be useful for understanding or changing how I am?

  Yes ☐ No ☐

- Is a specific task so that I will know when I have done it?

  Yes ☐ No ☐

- Is realistic, practical and achievable?

  Yes ☐ No ☐

- Makes clear what I am going to do and when I am going to do it.

  Yes ☐ No ☐

- Is an activity that won't be easily blocked or prevented by practical problems?

  Yes ☐ No ☐

- Will help me to learn useful things even if it doesn't work out perfectly?

  Yes ☐ No ☐

Remember to review your progress in making these changes weekly, and to make sure the changes are practical and achievable.

My notes

My Irritability diary

Date and time	Record your recent sleep/drink and feelings of pressure leading up to irritation	People and events leading up to feeling irritable	My feelings at the time	My thoughts at the time	Altered physical symptoms	My altered behaviour
	– Are you feeling tired? – Have you been drinking alcohol or caffeine? – Are you feeling pressured or hassled leading up to the time you felt annoyed?	– Where were you? – Who were you with? – What were you doing? – What was said/happened?	How did you feel emotionally at the time? – Were you irritable, annoyed or angry? – Any other emotions (anxious, ashamed depressed or guilty)?	– Any thoughts about: – Things not being fair? – Being picked on or mocked? – Being ignored? – Or about: – How you are coping? – The worst that could happen? – How others see you? – Your own body, behaviour or performance? – Any memories or mental pictures?	Note down any strong physical symptoms you noticed at the time, e.g. tension, rapid heartbeat, breaking out in a sweat, breathing faster, feeling shaky.	– What did you do differently? – What did you say differently – and how did you say it? – Did you stop doing what you were doing, or start doing something different?

Overcoming Anxiety, Stress and Panic

A Five Areas Approach

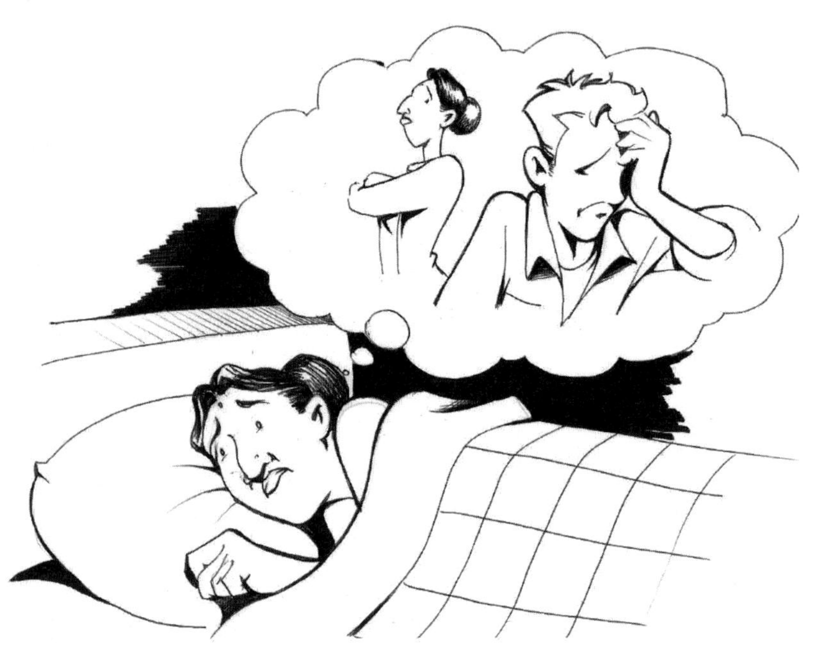

How to get a good night's sleep: overcoming anxiety and sleep problems

www.livinglifetothefull.com
www.fiveareas.com

Dr Chris Williams

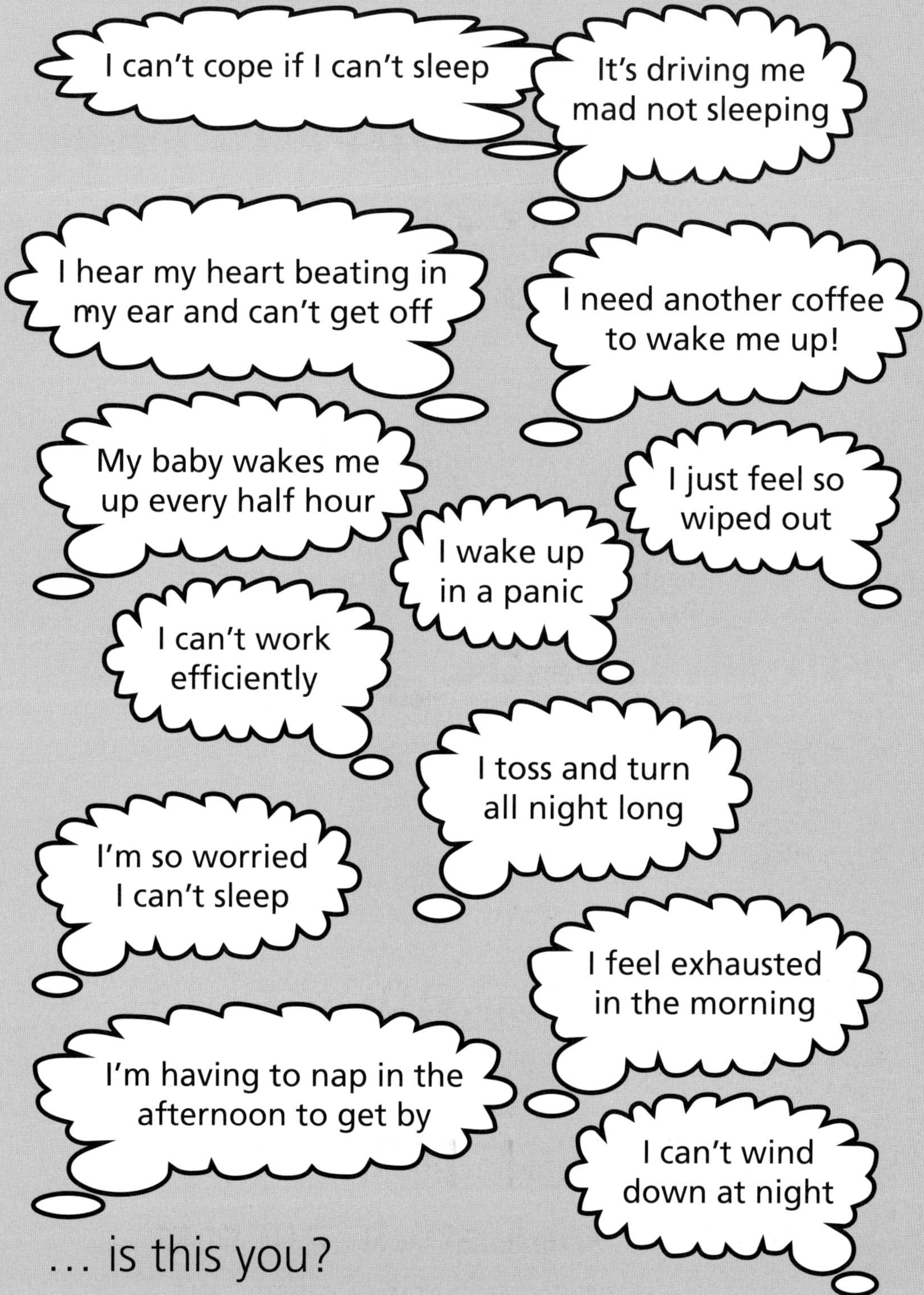
I can't cope if I can't sleep
It's driving me mad not sleeping
I hear my heart beating in my ear and can't get off
I need another coffee to wake me up!
My baby wakes me up every half hour
I just feel so wiped out
I wake up in a panic
I can't work efficiently
I toss and turn all night long
I'm so worried I can't sleep
I feel exhausted in the morning
I'm having to nap in the afternoon to get by
I can't wind down at night

… is this you?

If so … this **workbook is for you**.

In this workbook you will:

- Learn about sleep and sleeplessness.
- Learn about some common causes of sleep problems.
- Discover how stress and anxiety can affect sleep.
- Learn how to record your sleep pattern and identify things that worsen your sleep.
- Learn about making some changes that will help you sleep better.

What is enough sleep?

How much sleep you need varies from person to person. Some people feel well after sleeping only four to six hours a day, whereas others need as many as 10 or 12 hours a day. Both extremes are quite normal. What matters more is when your usual sleep pattern changes and you feel worse because of it.

What causes sleeplessness?

Most people have problems sleeping from time to time. Sleep problems often are caused by some stressful situation or life event, or they can be a result of your lifestyle.

Anxiety and stress are very common causes of sleeplessness – and so are other feelings such as depression, anger, guilt, shame and stress. In this workbook you will find out more about how all of them affect your sleep.

A Five Areas assessment of sleeplessness

Let's start by thinking about how sleeplessness is affecting you in five key areas of your life.

Area 1: People and events around you

Problems with noise

Noises that vary or come out of the blue can wake you from sleep. If you are feeling anxious and stressed, you may end up waking with a start, or tossing and turning in bed seething at the noise. Rather than just lying in bed feeling stressed, angry or got at, try tackling the problem. For example if you have noisy neighbours, could you or someone else ask them to turn down their television or music? Have you thought about fitting double-glazing or plastic sheeting inside windows to reduce noise? This needn't be expensive and many reasonably priced options are available. You can buy moulded ear plugs from your chemist.

Q Are there any sources of noise you can easily change?

Yes ☐ No ☐ Sometimes ☐

Your physical environment

- If your mattress is quite old, can you turn it over, rotate it or perhaps even change it? You may be able to add extra support, such as a board or old door underneath it.
- If your bedroom is too hot, try opening a window or using a fan. If it's too cold, think about using an extra blanket or duvet. Or you could think about insulation, draught excluders, secondary or double-glazing, or turning up the heat in the room.
- Is there too much light in the room? If bright lights such as streetlights come through your curtains, then consider the thickness of your curtains. Have you thought about adding a thicker lining or blackout lining? If this may not be possible, for example because of the cost involved, a black plastic bin bag can work well as a blackout blind. It can be stapled or stuck to the curtain rail or window surround. If you use sticky Velcro, you can easily put this up at night and take it down during the day.

Area 2: Your thinking

Worrying or anxious thoughts are a common cause of sleeplessness. Usually as you try to sleep, your tension levels go down. So your body and brain begin to relax and you drop off to sleep. But when you're anxious or worried, your brain becomes overly alert. You end up mulling over things again and again, for example, worrying that you may have upset someone. This is the exact opposite of what's needed to go to sleep. Worrying thoughts are therefore both a cause and effect of poor sleep.

You may have anxious thoughts or worries about:

- Life in general – for example, a stressful event such as an exam or interview, or a stressful situation such as not being able to pay a bill, or keeping a hospital or court appointment.
- Not sleeping – for example, about the fact you aren't sleeping and that this will cause you problems the next day.

When you think like this, your fears get blown out of proportion, for example, that your brain or your body will be harmed by lack of sleep. These fears prevent you going off to sleep.

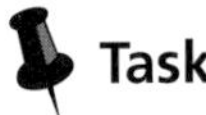

Do you worry about things in general or about not getting off to sleep?

Yes ☐ No ☐ Sometimes ☐

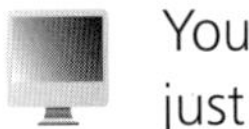

Task

If you answered 'Yes' or 'Sometimes', write down your worries on a sheet of paper or on a Worry strip.

You can download Worry strips for free from **www.fiveareas.com** – or just use a diary or a piece of paper.

Keep the Worry strip by your bed. Mark on it a **day and time** when you will spend time thinking through your worries and sorting out a plan of action. Plan to do your worrying later rather than now, while you are in bed. Use that time to also plan how you will sort out any problems. The *How to start fixing problems and finding solutions (practical problem solving)* workbook will be helpful here.

Training your mind to master anxious thoughts

Do you have so many worries that you can't imagine fixing them all? Is there so much to be concerned about that you feel overwhelmed? Do you ever feel panicky and get terrified about what might happen?

When you sit down to think through what you have written on your worry strips, you can also start to tackle your worries. Try the following steps:

1. Label it – for example: Oh you're just one of those worrying thoughts.
2. Leave it – worrying thoughts want attention, so try not to give them any.
3. Stand up to it – worrying thoughts are like bullies, weak underneath. You can beat them.
4. Give yourself a break – what would someone who really loved you say? Trust them and let them help you beat the bad thought.
5. Look at it differently – give yourself the advice you'd give to a friend. Ask yourself if it will matter in six months. Pick someone you know and work out how they would handle the situation. Trust the facts, not the worrying feelings.

The *Noticing and changing anxious thinking* workbook will help you practise using this approach.

How much sleep do you need?

By choosing to write down the worry on a Worry strip and put it off to a later time you can also test whether your fears are true or out of all proportion. The break in the cycle of thoughts gives your mind a rest. On thinking again, often you will discover that although you may feel tired, your fears that the very worst will happen don't usually come true.

It's helpful also to know that research shows that most people don't need very much sleep at all to be physically and mentally healthy. When people who describe poor sleep are asked to try to sleep in a sleep research laboratory, they often sleep far more than they think.

It's helpful to know that it is possible to function well with very little sleep each night.

Q Do you have extreme fears about the effect of not sleeping?

Yes ☐ No ☐ Sometimes ☐

Extreme (catastrophic) fears can themselves prevent you from falling asleep. You might feel tired and irritable the next day. But this doesn't necessarily affect your ability to do things around the house or at work.

Area 3: Your feelings (emotions)

Many strong feelings such as extreme worry or anxiety can be linked to sleeplessness.

Q Do you feel anxious when you try to sleep?

Yes ☐ No ☐ Sometimes ☐

If you answered 'Yes' or 'Sometimes', remember that anxiety is a common cause of sleeplessness. It often triggers your body's fear response causing adrenaline to flow. Adrenaline is a substance produced by your body that makes you feel fidgety or restless. Your anxiety therefore acts to keep you alert. This is the opposite of what you want when you're trying to fall asleep.

Check the relaxation modules available at **www.livinglifetothefull.com** and **www.fiveareas.com**.

Q Do you ever wake up feeling panicky with a racing heart or feeling breathless?

Yes ☐ No ☐ Sometimes ☐

Panic attacks can occur at night – especially if you have low mood. If this happens to you, it's important to know what is going on. Breathlessness can also be a symptom of heart problems, so it is important to check with your doctor what the cause is. If you know that the cause is panic try to:

1. Sit on the side of the bed.
2. Close your mouth.
3. Take normal-sized breaths.
4. Relax and drop your shoulders.

Remind yourself it is just panic and will settle soon. Once it does, lie down again and go back to sleep.

Q Are you feeling depressed, upset or low in mood and do you no longer enjoy things as before?

Yes ☐ No ☐ Sometimes ☐

If you answered 'Yes' or 'Sometimes', remember that depression is a common cause of sleeplessness. For example, when you are feeling depressed you may find that it takes you several hours to get to sleep. You may wake up several hours earlier than normal feeling unrested or on edge. Having treatment for your depression can often be helpful for improving your sleep.

Other feelings such as shame, guilt and anger can also cause sleeplessness.

Area 4: Altered physical symptoms

Pain, itching, breathlessness or other physical symptoms can cause sleeplessness. Tackling these physical symptoms will help with your sleep problems.

Q Do you ever notice your heart beating loudly in your ear?

Yes ☐ No ☐ Sometimes ☐

This is a common and normal event. If you turn over and find another body position, it will settle down.

Q Are other physical symptoms keeping you awake?

Yes ☐ No ☐ Sometimes ☐

If you answered 'Yes' or 'Sometimes', you should see your doctor as you may need medical treatment for your symptoms. If you have a heart condition and take water tablets, changing the timing may help. Taking these during the day rather than just before going to sleep can help stop you having to get up again and again to go the toilet. Once you have been checked physically by your doctor and are taking any appropriate treatments, then you can try out the various hints and tips that follow to help you cope with these different common sleep problems.

Area 5: Altered behaviour: unhelpful behaviours

Preparing for sleep

The time leading up to sleep is very important. Try to build in a '**wind-down**' time in the evening when you are less active and doing less stimulating activity. Physical over-activity such as exercising, eating too much, using the computer or watching TV just before going to bed can keep you awake. Sometimes people watch TV while lying in bed. This may help them wind down, but many people become more alert. So doing this adds to their sleep problems.

Q Are you doing things in bed which wake you up?

Yes ☐ No ☐ Sometimes ☐

If you answered 'Yes' or 'Sometimes', keep your bed as a place for sleep and for sex. Don't lie on your bed watching TV, or working or worrying. This will only wake you up and prevent you sleeping. You'll also need to decide whether listening to a radio or music helps you go to sleep.

What about caffeine?

Caffeine is a chemical found in cola drinks, coffee, tea, chocolate and some herbal drinks. It causes you to be more alert. People who have lots of caffeine for several weeks can get addicted to it. It also reduces your sleep quality.

There is a risk of getting caught in a vicious circle – in which tiredness causes you to drink more caffeine to keep alert. Then the caffeine itself affects your sleep and worsens the original tiredness. Try not to drink more than five cups of strong coffee or equivalent in one day.

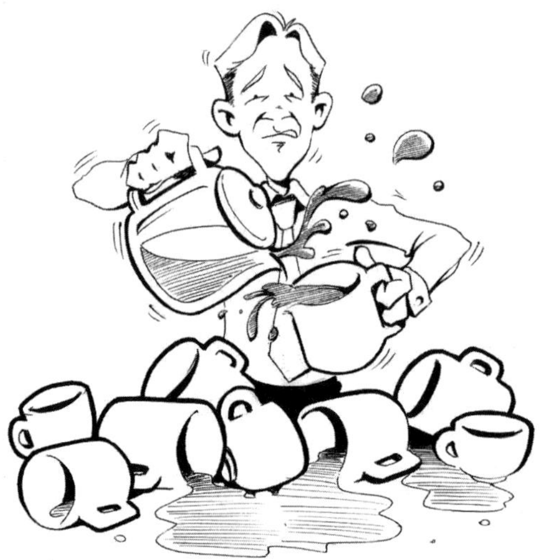

Key point

Caffeine stays in your body for a few hours before it is broken down inside your body and leaves in your urine. This means that you should avoid drinking caffeine-containing drinks in the few hours leading up to bed.

Q Are you taking too much caffeine?

Yes ☐ No ☐ Sometimes ☐

If you answered 'Yes' or 'Sometimes', you should reduce the amount of caffeine-containing drinks you take. Do this in a step-by-step way, for example by switching slowly to decaffeinated cola, coffee or tea. Some people find that a warm milky drink can help them fall asleep.

What about alcohol?

Sometimes people drink alcohol to reduce their feelings of tension and to help them get off to sleep. But drinking alcohol can actually cause problems, such as anxiety, depression and sleeplessness. Also, drinking too much may cause you to go to the toilet more than usual. This can also keep you awake.

Q Are you drinking too much alcohol?

Yes ☐ No ☐ Sometimes ☐

If you answered 'Yes' or 'Sometimes', you can use the workbook *Stress, alcohol and drugs*, to plan to cut down in a slow, step-by-step manner. Discuss how best to do this with your GP or healthcare worker.

What about your sleep pattern?

If you aren't sleeping well, you can be tempted to go to bed either much earlier or much later than normal or to nap during the day.

Q Do you have a disrupted sleep pattern (time to bed/getting up)?

Yes ☐ No ☐ Sometimes ☐

If you answered 'Yes' or 'Sometimes', you need to set yourself regular sleep times. A regular sleep pattern can help to maintain a clear start and end to the day. Try therefore to get up between 7 a.m. and 9 a.m. and to sleep between about 11 p.m. and midnight. Adjust these times to fit your own circumstances.

Try to avoid daytime napping. Napping disrupts your natural sleep–wake cycle. By doing this, you will teach your body what time to fall asleep and what time to get up.

If you have a baby

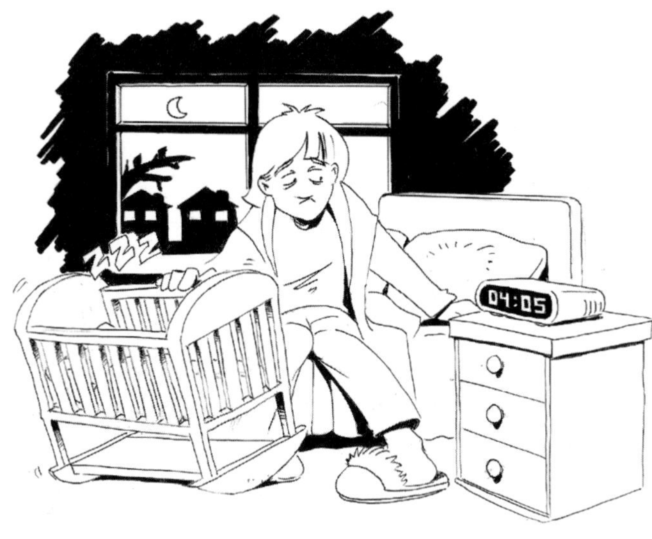

A major cause of sleeplessness is having a baby in the house. It may take a baby several months or even longer to sleep through the night. Also, feeding during the night disrupts your sleep pattern until your baby is old enough to eat or drink enough to see them through the night.

The Secrets of the Baby Whisperer: How to Calm, Connect and Communicate with Your Baby by Tracy Hogg is a widely recommended book for people with babies. You may find this book helpful to establish a regular sleeping pattern for your baby – and help teach them ways of settling and soothing themselves. You can order the book from any bookshop or from **www.fiveareas.com**.

As a practical solution, if your baby wakes up often during the night and sleeps during the day, it's understandable to take some sleep when you can. When your baby starts to settle into a more regular sleep–wake cycle, it is a good time for you to then cut down on your own daytime sleeps.

Tossing and turning in bed and clock watching

Q Do you find yourself lying awake in bed tossing and turning, waking your partner up to talk ('Are you awake ... ?'), or just watching the clock?

Yes ☐ No ☐ Sometimes ☐

If you answered 'Yes' or 'Sometimes', then some practical changes can help, such as moving the clock so you can't see it. It can still be in the room so that you can set an alarm or reach it if you have to.

Keeping a sleep diary

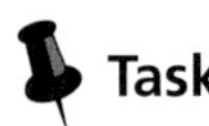

Task

You may find it helpful to use a **Sleep diary** for a few days this week. A blank sleep diary is included at the end of this workbook. You can copy out the headings or photocopy the diary. By completing the diary you will be able to identify what important factors affect your sleep.

Carrying out your own Five Areas assessment

Look at the Five Areas assessment in the figure below. Write in all the things you have identified that affect your sleep. These will be your possible targets for change.

Five Areas assessment of factors affecting my sleep

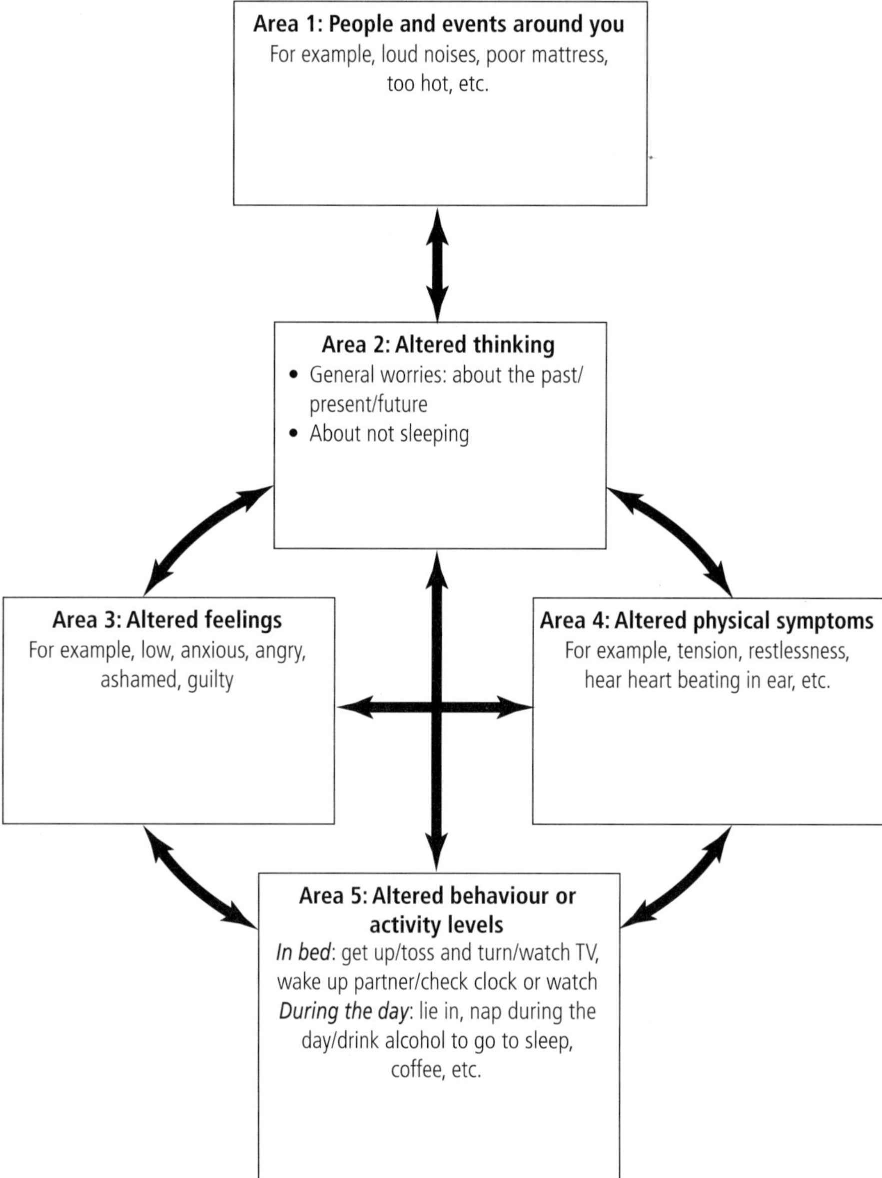

Overcoming sleeplessness

Use the checklist below to find out about things you can do to get rid of your sleep problems.

Sleep checklist: Some things to do and not do

Some things to do in the run up to bed and during the day	Tick here if this affects your life – even if just sometimes	Some changes you can make and resources you can use
Plan a wind-down time each evening	☐	Having a warm, bran-based milky drink may help. Think about having a bath and listening to relaxing music. If you like candles or scented oils try using those
Have a regular time to go to bed and to get up	☐	To help you get back into a routine
Tackle the things that you know affect your sleep environment (for example external noise, mattress)	☐	See earlier in this workbook (pages 155–6). If your neighbours cause the noise, the *How to start fixing problems and finding solutions (practical problem solving)* and *How to ask for what you really need (being assertive)* workbooks will help you find ways of dealing with this problem. Plan changes to your room/bed as needed
Reduce your general life pressures	☐	Say no – balance demands you put on yourself. Allow space and time for yourself. The *How to ask for what you really need (being assertive)* workbook can help you with this
Stop, think and reflect on worrying thoughts about the past, the present and the future, and also about sleep	☐	If worrying thoughts keep you awake, write down your worries on a piece of paper or on a Worry strip (from **www.fiveareas.com**). Decide to think through your worries properly at a planned time on one of the coming few days. Use the *Noticing and changing anxious thinking* workbook to put your thoughts into perspective, or the *How to start fixing problems and finding solutions (practical problem solving)* workbook to tackle things that need to change
Live reasonably healthily. People who are fitter generally sleep better	☐	It might sound strange to say this, but over-doing healthy living may become unhealthy, for example doing too much exercise. Try to live healthily but not obsessively so
Use relaxation tapes or techniques if you find them helpful	☐	You may wish to try the free downloadable relaxation MP3 resources at **www.livinglifetothefull.com** and **www.fiveareas.com**, using Anxiety Control Training (originally developed by Dr Philip Snaith)
Avoid drinking too much alcohol or caffeine (or smoking) just before bed	☐	Alcohol causes sleep to be shallow and unrefreshing. It can also make you wake up more to use the toilet. Also watch out for cola drinks, or too much coffee, tea or hot chocolate, which contain caffeine. Try a planned switch to decaffeinated drinks or water. Don't smoke just before going to bed as this can cause sleeplessness too
Avoid doing things that stimulate you mentally or physically in the run-up to sleep (for example using the computer,or watching an exciting film).	☐	You can of course do all these things, but stop doing them at least an hour before going to bed. Avoid doing them in bed too
Don't respond in ways that end up backfiring or worsening things (for example lying in during the day, napping beyond the time it's helpful)	☐	Try to re-set your body clock by getting up at a set time each day. Try to avoid napping and go to bed at roughly the same time each day to get into a regular routine
Don't look for answers to sleeplessness in sleeping tablets	☐	These tablets are not advisable in the long term

Don't expect to change everything immediately. But with practice, you can make helpful changes to your sleep pattern. If you find it hard at first, just do what you can.

Your own Five Areas assessment may have helped you identify the problems you have at present. The table above will have provided you with hints and tips in each of your main problem areas.

Summary

In this workbook you have learnt about:

- Sleep and sleeplessness.
- Some common causes of sleep problems.
- How stress and anxiety can affect sleep.
- How to record your sleep pattern and identify things that worsen your sleep.
- Making some changes that will help you sleep better.

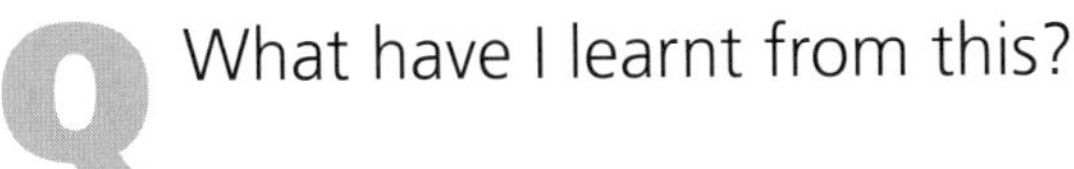

What have I learnt from this?

Q What do I want to try *next*?

Putting what you have learned into practice

Look back at the **Sleep checklist of things to do and not do** on page 166. Plan to make changes in how you prepare for sleep and what you do once you are in bed.

Write down what you're going to do this week, to put into practice what you have learnt.

My practice plan

What changes am I going to make?

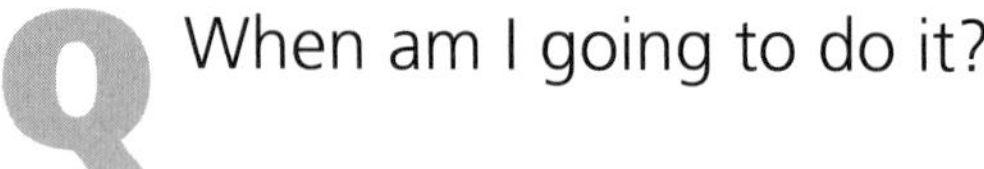

When am I going to do it?

Q What problems could arise, and how can I sort these?

Apply the **Questions for effective change** to your plan.

Q Is my planned task one that:

- Will be useful for understanding or changing how I am?

  Yes ☐ No ☐

- Is a specific task so that I will know when I have done it?

  Yes ☐ No ☐

- Is realistic, practical and achievable?

  Yes ☐ No ☐

- Makes clear what I am going to do and when I am going to do it.

  Yes ☐ No ☐

- Is an activity that won't be easily blocked or prevented by practical problems?

  Yes ☐ No ☐

- Will help me to learn useful things even if it doesn't work out perfectly?

  Yes ☐ No ☐

Remember to review your progress in making these changes weekly, and to make sure the changes are practical and achievable.

My notes

My Sleep diary

Time when you are in bed and trying to sleep	Record when you are asleep with an 'X'	When in bed, record any thoughts/images that go through your mind and keep you awake (for example worries, fears about sleeping or the effect of not sleeping). Write them on piece of paper or your Worry strip	Record any activities you do that relate to sleep. *Before bed*: alcohol, caffeine, smoking, exercise, daytime napping, computer games, watching scary films, sleeping in. *In bed*: reading, listening to the radio, disturbing other people, tossing/turning, getting up and going downstairs, etc.
8.00 p.m.– 9.59 p.m.			
10.00 p.m. – 11.59 p.m.			
12.00 a.m. – 1.59 a.m.			
2.00 a.m. – 3.59 a.m.			
4.00 a.m. – 5.59 a.m.			
6.00 a.m. – 7.59 a.m.			
8.00 a.m. – 9.59 a.m.			
10.00 a.m. – 11.59 a.m.			
12.00 p.m. – 1.59 p.m.			
2.00 p.m. – 3.59 p.m.			
4.00 p.m. – 5.59 p.m.			
6.00 p.m. — 7.59 p.m.			

Overcoming Anxiety, Stress and Panic

A Five Areas Approach

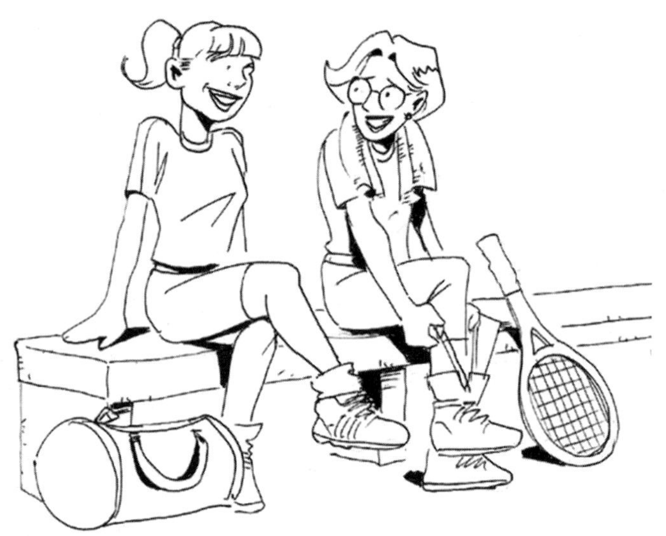

Using exercise to overcome stress

www.livinglifetothefull.com
www.fiveareas.com

Dr Chris Williams

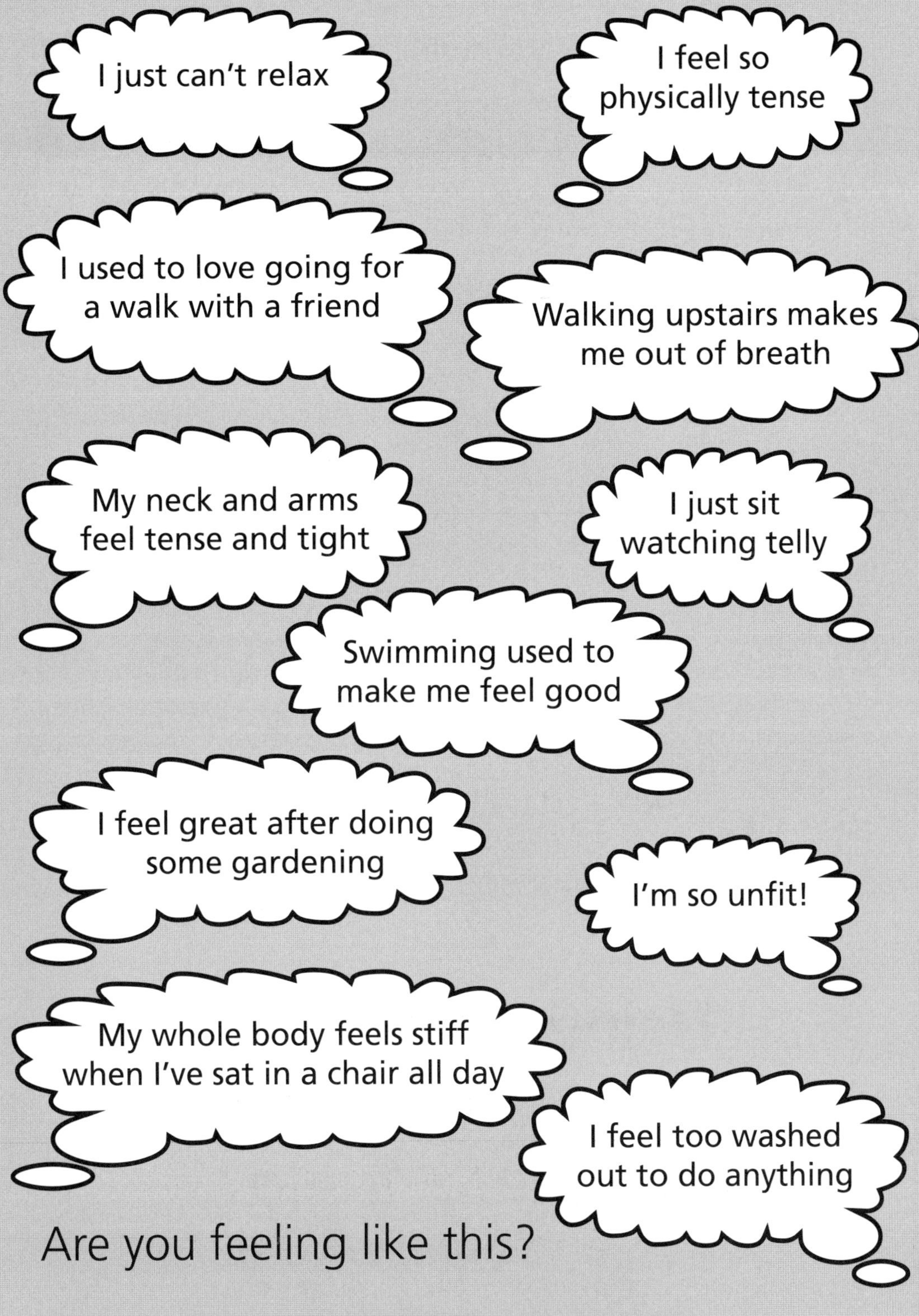

Are you feeling like this?

If so ... this **workbook is for you**.

In this workbook you will:

- See how exercise can boost your mood and help you relax.
- Learn how to plan exercise to reduce your tension and anxiety.
- Discover how exercise can help you feel fitter, more active and better about yourself.

Why bother with exercise?

As your mind and body affect each other, when you feel anxious and mentally tense, you also feel tense physically. For example you may feel restless and unable to relax. Mental tension can also cause physical tension in your muscles and joints. So you may feel shaky or have pain, weakness or tiredness. It can be surprising how tiring anxiety can be. Some people may feel completely exhausted when they have felt anxious for a time. Their muscles are so tense it can seem as if they have run a marathon all day.

Now think back to a time when you exercised – such as riding a bike, running or swimming. Some people find that they often get a **mental 'high'** after exercise. They feel more relaxed both mentally and physically. Exercising in the day can also help you relax at night and sleep better as well.

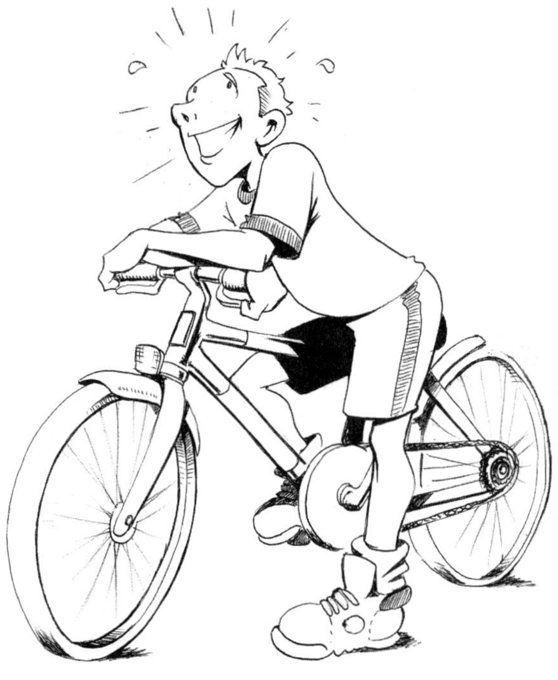

By **increasing your physical activity levels, you can boost how you feel** mentally as well as physically. This will also help you feel more relaxed as well.

Why exercise may be good for you

People often forget to exercise when they feel stressed. It may seem you are working hard just to survive or get by, or it just seems too hard to do. But exercise has been shown to be a helpful part of a treatment course for stress and anxiety. You can also choose to 'prescribe' exercise for yourself as part of your own self-treatment plan.

- Exercise can be fun if you choose something that you have previously liked doing.
- Self-treatment gives **you** control to plan things at your own pace.
- It can help you structure and plan your day – rather than just staying in and being inactive.
- Exercise can boost your social life. Doing things with others such as a step class, playing football or going for a swim can help you meet others with a shared interest.
- Even with a baby you can think of ways to exercise. Check out whether there are any aqua-aerobics or mother/baby exercise and massage classes in your area.
- And if you have a baby or toddler, walking with the pram (and another mum or dad) is also good exercise.

It really is a win–win situation.

Are there any downsides of exercise?

- If you are physically unwell, you may not be able to do certain exercises for a time. Ask your doctor or health visitor for advice about what you can or can't do if you are ill or have had a recent operation.
- You may have aching muscles to begin with (the author does!).
- There can be a cost for some activities (for example, for using a gym or a swimming pool).

How planned exercise can help you feel better

Experiment

You'll need less than 15 minutes to do this experiment. The aim is to test if even a small amount of exercise affects how you feel overall.

Before you start think of a physical activity that you can do. This should be something:

- That is realistic, bearing in mind how you are physically at the moment.
- That can be done in just 5–10 minutes to start with.
- You know is within your capabilities and doesn't push you.

Here's an example: walk up and down a flight of stairs three to four times. Take rest in between if you get out of breath.

Key point

Aim to do something that gets your heart rate up and gets you moving **without being excessive**. You aren't being asked to do a workout. You don't need to get changed, work up a sweat or even do warm-up exercises!

Other things you could try are stretching your body, jogging slowly on the spot or walking round the block at a reasonable pace. If you have a small child, you can do the last one with your child in a pram.

Remember:

- Not to overdo it – exercise is good in moderate amounts.
- If you think you're physically unwell you can always check this with your doctor first.
- Any benefits can be boosted even more by planning to do activities that are fun or sociable.

Doing your planned exercise

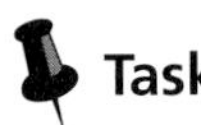

Task

So now you've chosen what to do. **Before you start** put a cross on the two lines below to show how you feel right now.

How I feel now

Before your exercise

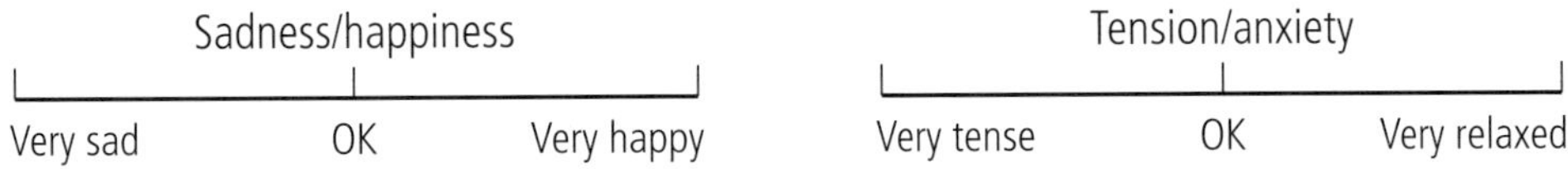

Now do your 5–10 minutes of light exercise. Remember you can stop for a rest if you feel this is too long for you. **Immediately afterwards** rate your mood again.

Your review

After your exercise

Next: stop, think and reflect

Have a look at your scores before and after.

Q Did you notice any changes? Write down any changes you noticed in your thoughts/mental energy/how positive you feel/your ability to think clearly:

Q How did you feel during the task? Write down how you felt emotionally (tension, anger, stress, sadness, happiness, enthusiasm):

Q How did you feel physically? Write down here how you felt physically (relaxed/tense, jittery, tired, achy, ready for more):

Write down any other changes you noticed:

Overall, do you think you might benefit from planning some exercise into your life as part of your own 'mental fitness' package?

Yes ☐ No ☐ Yes, but… ☐

Yes, but …

Remember, often people know there are lots of things in life that are good for them, but they don't do them. That's just as true in other people's lives as it may be in your own.

Tackling the simple blocks

Many people see exercise as too hard or boring, too expensive, taking too much time – or all of these! Often the biggest problems are simple ones:

- Perhaps you just aren't in the habit of doing exercise.
- Or maybe you want to get into the habit of doing exercise but you think it will be too hard. For example, it's easy for people to talk themselves out of it. This is a common problem.

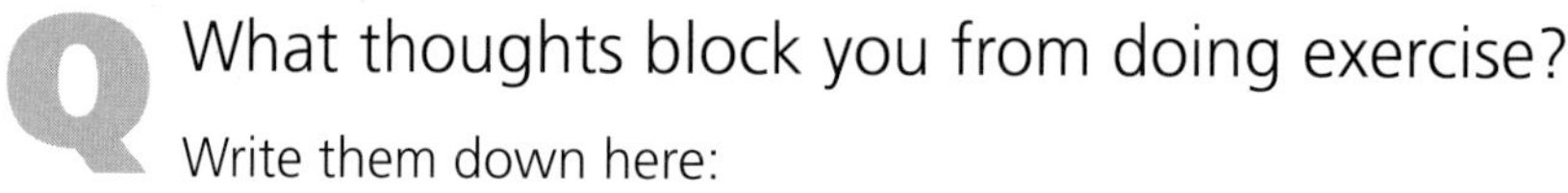

Q What thoughts block you from doing exercise?

Write them down here:

Well done! Now that you know what's blocking you from doing exercise you can work to overcome it.

Remember that planning to do exercise doesn't mean you have to make a big change to your lifestyle. Even **small changes** can make a positive difference. So aim to find a way to make this easier for yourself, for example, fitting it into what you already do each day.

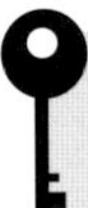

Key point

Exercise and injury: Remember it's important to **warm up to avoid muscle pulls, aches and strains**. Using good techniques and the right equipment, clothing and shoes is also important.

Planning when and how to exercise

People are often amazed at how empowering, energising and relaxing doing some regular exercise can be. It can boost your mood, and help you to relax your mind and body.

- Choose something that gets you going physically.
- Build up the amount of exercise slowly in a gradual and planned way.
- Don't throw yourself into things too quickly (or start too slowly): **pacing is the key**.
- Many people find that doing exercise towards the start of the day helps them to 'get going'.
- Avoid exercising just before going to bed as this can unhelpfully affect your sleep.
- Look to do this with help. Plan to exercise with a friend or relative. This has the added benefit of encouraging you to go if you find it's difficult (to avoid letting them down). And there's another big bonus as well – that you are doing something with someone, chatting and talking as you do it. This will help boost your **sense of closeness**, which again will also help your mood.
- Remember that walking with your children or partner or a friend, talking to them about what you see as you walk, is a good example of cheap and effective exercise.
- If you have a partner then remember that sex can be a great way of getting active, using calories, as well as building your relationship. Some people say it can be fun too.

It is often helpful to actively plan exercise into your day and diary rather than just 'trying to fit it in sometime'. You may find the following **planning task** helpful in making this regular commitment.

My plan to use exercise to help me feel better

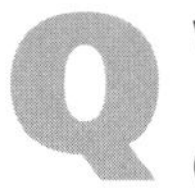

What am I going to do?

(Remember to choose something that is possible, realistic and achievable. Preferably choose something that is fun. Think about planning some exercise that has a social aspect at least once a week, for example walking with a friend, a step or yoga class or going for a run or walk with others. Remember exercise doesn't need to cost lots of money. You can get exercise videos and DVDs for a small weekly charge from your local library. Or you could walk to your local shop each time instead of taking the bus or being driven.)

When am I going to plan to do some exercise?

(Think if doing some exercise every day is practical for you. If it is, what time of day would be best for you? If you can't manage it every day then how about just once or twice a week? You can always build upon this at a later stage.)

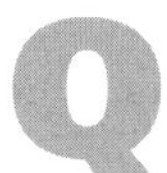

How much exercise will I do?

(Be realistic – think about your current level of fitness, health and motivation. If you have doubts about your health, please discuss this with your doctor.)

Q Is this **realistic**, practical and achievable?

(You know your own life and its various demands and commitments.)

Q What problems could prevent me doing this, and how can I overcome them?

(For example your daily routine, work or family deadlines such as picking up children from school, money, or having the kit you need.)

Keeping on track

Once you have created your exercise plan it is **important to keep on track**. This means setting yourself goals and reviewing your progress. In this way you can make changes if things aren't going well.

My plan for the next few weeks

Think about changes you want to make:

- In the short term (where you want to be in a few weeks time).
- In the medium-term (where you want to be in a few months time).
- In the long-term (where you want to be in a year's time).

Date of my next review

(Review your plan monthly, set aside a time to do this. Put it into your schedule or diary.)

Summary

In this workbook you have learned:

- How exercise can boost your mood and help you relax.
- How to plan exercise to reduce your tension and anxiety.
- How exercise can help you feel fitter, more active and better about yourself.

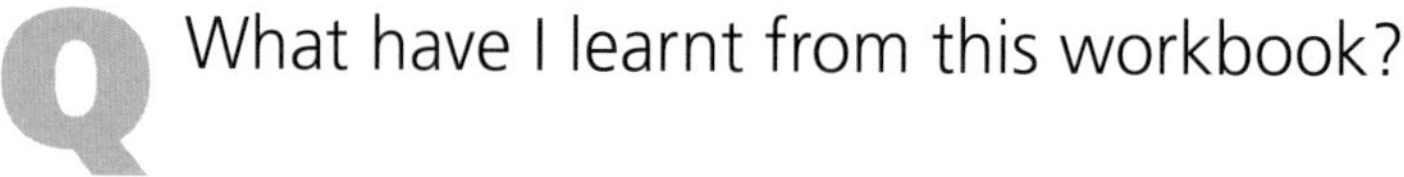

What have I learnt from this workbook?

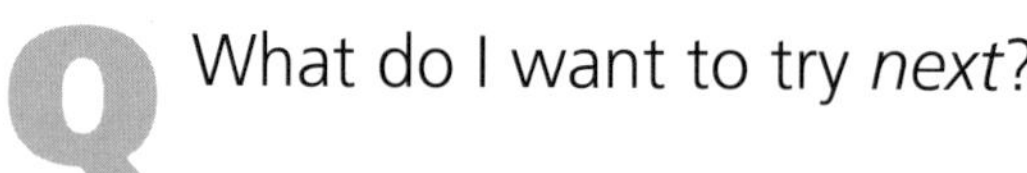

What do I want to try *next*?

Putting things into practice

Read this workbook again and then plan your own exercise. Try to stick to your plan.

Other sources of support

- Look out for classes at your local swimming pool or gym. Some pools and gyms also have crèches or clubs for babies or children.
- Think about tennis, badminton or walking classes.
- Do it with a friend! Plan to do exercise with a friend or colleague.

Do the online TV module about healthy living at **www.livinglifetothefull.com**. You can download free Mood Cards to rate your mood before and after exercise from **www.fiveareas.com**.

My notes

Overcoming Anxiety, Stress and Panic

A Five Areas Approach

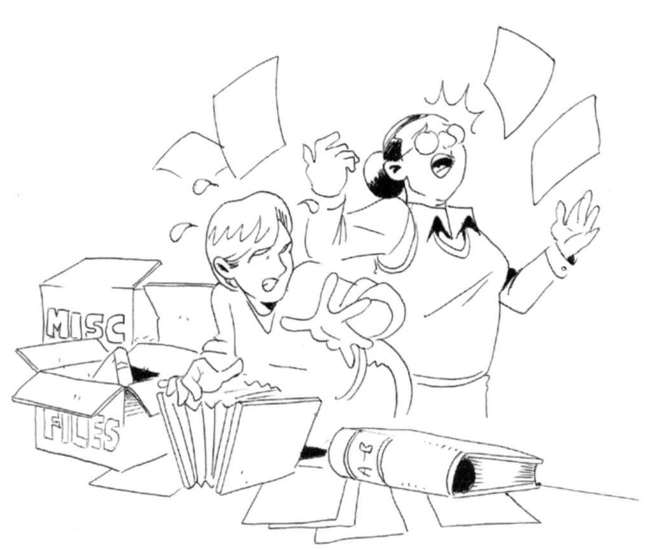

Things you do that worsen your anxiety (unhelpful behaviours)

www.livinglifetothefull.com
www.fiveareas.com

Dr Chris Williams

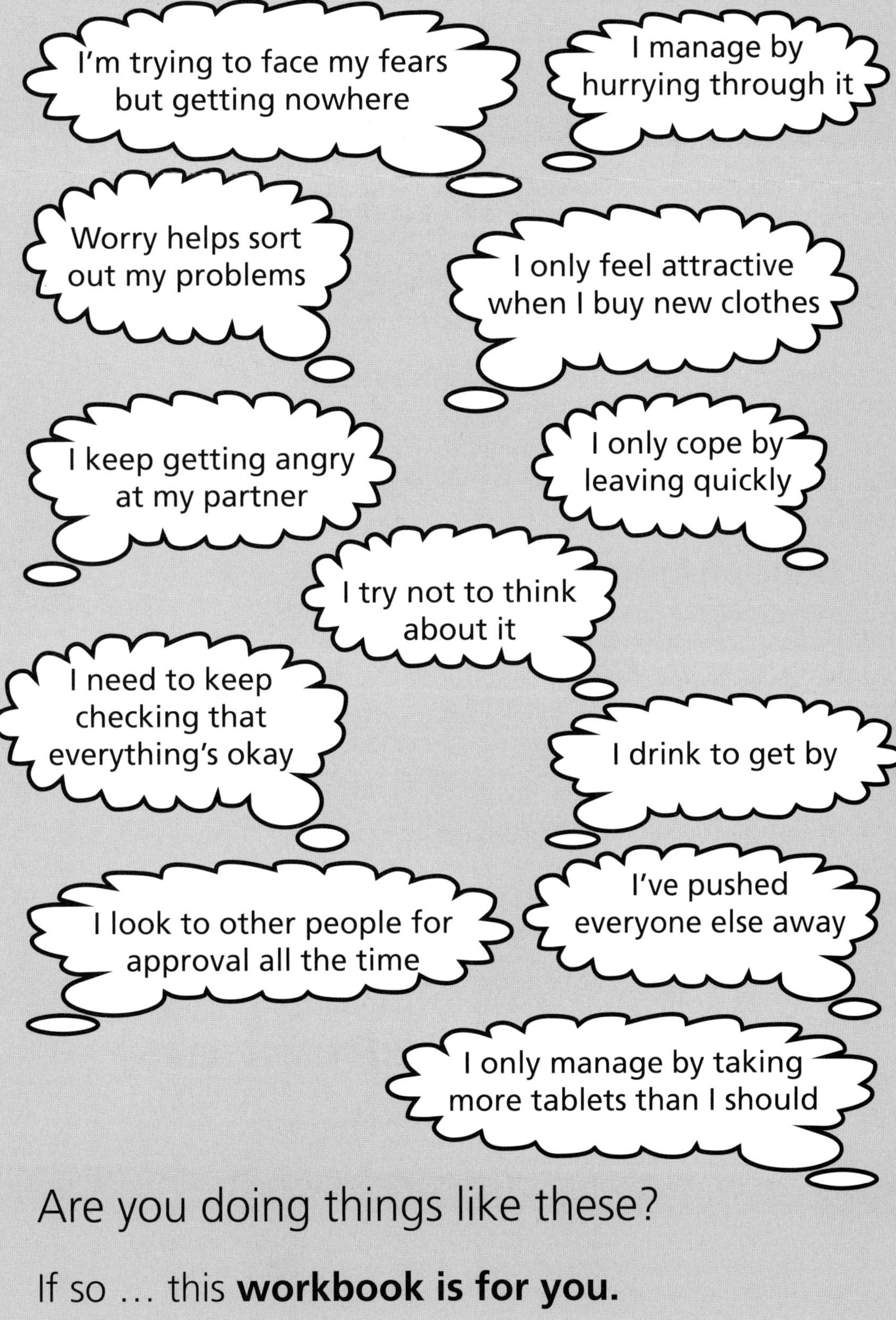
I'm trying to face my fears but getting nowhere
I manage by hurrying through it
Worry helps sort out my problems
I only feel attractive when I buy new clothes
I keep getting angry at my partner
I only cope by leaving quickly
I try not to think about it
I need to keep checking that everything's okay
I drink to get by
I look to other people for approval all the time
I've pushed everyone else away
I only manage by taking more tablets than I should

Are you doing things like these?

If so … this **workbook is for you.**

In this workbook you will:

- Discover how some things you do can prevent you tackling anxiety.
- Find out about how some activities can actually make you feel worse.
- Learn some helpful ways to tackle unhelpful behaviours.
- Make a clear plan to reduce an unhelpful behaviour.
- Plan some next steps to build on this.

Helpful and unhelpful behaviours

When people feel distressed, it is normal to try to do things to feel better. But their responses may be *helpful* or *unhelpful*. Helpful behaviours include finding out more about problems, creating a clear plan for change and reviewing your progress.

Unhelpful behaviours

Examples of common unhelpful behaviours are:

- Getting angry at others.
- Pushing people away.
- Drinking too much to block how you feel.

These behaviours are unhelpful because of the effect they have on everyone. Getting angry can end up with you feeling alone. This can prevent you getting the help and support the other person would otherwise have offered. So both you and they feel worse as a result.

Why do unhelpful behaviours happen?

People tend to do unhelpful things simply because these actions can make them feel better – **in the short term**. However, they can also backfire and create more problems. So eventually, they become part of the problem.

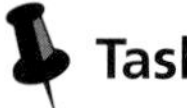
Task

Look at the following list and tick any activity that you did in the past few weeks. Many different unhelpful activities have been included in the list to help you to think about the unhelpful things that could be happening in your life.

Checklist: Identifying your unhelpful behaviour

As a result of how you feel, do you:	Tick here if you have noticed this – even if just sometimes
Eat too much to block how you feel ('comfort eating') or eat so much that this becomes a 'binge'?	☐
Make impulsive decisions about important things? For example, resigning a job without really thinking through the consequences	☐
Set yourself up to fail?	☐
Try to spend your way out of how you feel by going shopping ('retail therapy')?	☐
Watch TV programmes such as soaps or browse the internet, etc. to block how you feel – and act as substitutes for other relationships around you?	☐
Look to others to make decisions or sort out problems for you?	☐
Over-prepare and work really hard to prevent things going wrong?	☐
Set yourself up to be rejected by others?	☐
Throw yourself into doing things so that you are too busy to think about emotional or relationship issues?	☐
Not let others help you with things?	☐
Look to others to do everything you would normally do?	☐
Push others away by being verbally or physically rude to them?	☐
Deliberately harm yourself to block how you feel?	☐
Take risks, for example cross the road without looking, or gamble using money you don't have?	☐
Avoid having sex with your partner to get back at them or because you feel anxious, unattractive or angry?	☐
Check, clean or feel compelled to do things a set number of times or in exactly the 'correct' order so as to make things 'right'?	☐
Or do you spend a lot of time deliberately thinking 'good' thoughts to make things feel 'right' or counting good things you've done? (If you do this, you should see your doctor to discuss whether you may have a condition called obsessive-compulsive disorder.)	☐

In addition to the above, when you feel anxious, there are three more types of behaviour that can be especially important. These are behaviours that keep making you feel anxious and can stop you improving.

As a result of how you feel, do you:	Tick here if you have noticed this – even if just sometimes
1. Hurrying through things and trying to leave/escape quickly For example: walking or talking faster; cutting things short; making your excuses and leaving; or even lying that you need to be elsewhere or feel ill	☐
2. Doing things that make you feel safer in the short term For example: seeking constant reassurance from others; looking to others to make decisions for you, do things for you, or come along with you when you feel scared; or mis-using medication, drink or street drugs to give you false courage and block how you feel	☐
3. Trying hard to distract yourself from fearful or worrying thoughts or physical symptoms For example: trying to say positive comments again and again ('I'll be alright, I'll be alright'); trying to think hard of something else (such as counting the tiles on a wall); doing something physical to hurt or distract you from fears (such as clenching your fists, biting your lip, digging your nails into your hand)	☐

Key point

All the behaviours listed in the table – hurrying/escaping, trying to feel safe in unhelpful ways, and trying to distract yourself from fears – seem very helpful at the time. However, they are all ways of *subtle avoidance*. They make you feel better – but only at the time. In the long term, they can actually worsen how you feel.

Here is an example of how these behaviours can backfire.

Example: Sam's anxiety

Sam has been feeling very scared when she tries to teach in class. She feels she will mess it up and be humiliated. As a result she has spent a lot of time anxiously worrying about this. This has led her to spend many hours preparing presentations. She practises them again and again before she feels she can present something to her students. When she does a presentation that goes well, this teaches her the unhelpful rule that she has only just pulled it off, and that she must prepare even more next time.

But this backfires because it leaves her feeling stressed all the time. She also has little spare time at home. As a result, she has been arguing with her partner Andrea who thinks she needs to relax more. This is driving them apart as a couple and causing both of them to be upset. Sam's over-preparing for things is therefore backfiring for both of them.

So if you are using these behaviours, you need to become aware that they are unhelpful and tackle them as part of your problem. The main reasons why these behaviours are unhelpful are that:

- Their purpose is to block how you feel rather than stop you feeling anxious.
- They stop you doing the things you had actually wanted to do – they knock you off course.
- They teach you that the way to cope is by avoiding stressful situations. In fact, the opposite is true. Facing up to your worries and successfully tackling stress is the best solution.

Key point

Both *helpful* and *unhelpful* behaviours make you feel better in the short term. But the key difference between them is that in the longer term **unhelpful behaviours backfire**. They worsen how you or others feel. So they become part of your problem. The good news is that if this applies to you, you can make changes.

Write down any other unhelpful behaviours you've noticed doing:

Now think back on your answers.

Q Are some of your behaviours unhelpful in the short term or longer term either for you or for others around you?

Yes ☐ No ☐ Sometimes ☐

Choose just one example and write down its effect.

Effect on me:

Effect on others:

Unhelpful support from other people

Some people may offer 'helpful advice' all the time and want to do **everything** for you. There can be many reasons for this such as being concerned about you, friendship or love. Sometimes it may be because the other person feels anxious or even guilty about how you feel. Whatever the cause, when others offer too much help and want to do everything for you, their actions can backfire:

- You may feel suffocated and frustrated.
- You may feel treated like a child.
- Irritation may build up and upset both you and the other person.
- Their support may make you feel less confident.

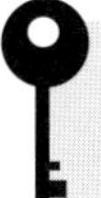

Key point

When trying to cope with stress and anxiety it's important that you continue to do as many things as you are able to do. If others take over too much responsibility from you, it can undermine your confidence rather than helping you feel better.

Similarly, looking to others for constant reassurance or to make all decisions for you also saps your confidence in the long term. Just as it isn't a good idea for teenage children to have everything done for them, the same is true of adults.

But there's good news. Discovering that unhelpful behaviours are part of what's keeping you feeling bad, means that you have now identified something you can change. By working through the seven steps described below you can learn an approach that will help you change any unhelpful behaviour.

Overcoming your own unhelpful behaviour

Step 1: Identify and clearly define the unhelpful behaviour

Did you tick several boxes in the checklist on page 187? The first thing to do is to choose just one unhelpful behaviour to change.

Choosing a first target

Example: Sam's target

Sam decides she wants to change her habit of over-preparing for her classes.

Now, write down one single unhelpful behaviour that you want to change here:

Be a detective

The next thing is to do some research on your behaviour. First, record your unhelpful behaviour over several days. Make a written note of:

- When it occurs.
- How much and how often you do it (for example, how much preparation did you do, how much did you drink, how many times you've sought reassurance, how often have you hurried away etc.).
- How long it lasts for.

Use the **diary** at the end of this workbook to help you understand more about your unhelpful behaviour. Try to work out what it may be that affects how you respond at the time. For example:

- The time of day.
- Who you are with and how they responded.
- What went through your mind.
- How you felt emotionally and physically at the time.

- Any other things you tend to do to cope or escape.
- And anything else that seems to help explain your reaction.

Check point: Is your target a realistic target? Answer the **Questions for effective change** to find out:

Q Is your target:

- Clear and realistic and something that you can tackle over the next week or two?

  Yes ☐ No ☐

- Not so scary that you can't face doing it?

  Yes ☐ No ☐

- Something that will still help you move forwards?

  Yes ☐ No ☐

Key point

Sometimes you need to make sure that your first target really is a small, focused problem so that you can tackle it in one step.

Now use your diary to decide if you need to break down the unhelpful behaviour into smaller steps that you can target one at a time.

Q Do you need to break it down into a number of smaller more achievable targets?

Yes ☐ No ☐

If you answered 'No', then please go straight to Step 2. If you answered 'Yes', then read the example below about how to make sure you've chosen a realistic first target and write it down again. If you need to, write down your new smaller first target here.

Example: Sam breaks her target into smaller steps

Sam keeps a record of when she ends up over-preparing for classes. She realises that several things affect this. It's often when:

- She has slept poorly.
- It's an unfamiliar topic she hasn't taught before.
- She is teaching a class which has two 'difficult' boys in it – who snigger from time to time. She has difficulty dealing with them.

Sam realises there are three separate things here she could work on. She decides to first think about how she can tackle the two rude boys. She uses the *How to start fixing problems and finding solutions (practical problem solving)* workbook to get some ideas of what to do. She decides she will split them up by where they sit in the room, and also take them to one side with a colleague to discuss their progress. This works well and helps take some of the pressure off.

She then moves on to working through the *How to get a good night's sleep: overcoming anxiety and sleep problems* workbook. She finds this really helps – and finds she is far less irritable when she has slept better. This also helps her in how she gets on with Andrea. Finally, Sam returns to this workbook and decides to focus on how she can plan to limit the amount of preparation time to a sensible amount.

My clear first step is:

Remember this should be a small, focused problem you can tackle in one step.

Well done!

Step 2: Think up as many solutions as possible to stop your unhelpful behaviour

Now you need to come up with as many ideas as possible to tackle this first unhelpful behaviour. From among them you should be able to identity a realistic, practical and achievable solution.

Include completely whacky ideas in your list as well, even if you wouldn't choose to do them. This will help you to **think broadly**. Here are some useful questions to help you to think up possible solutions:

- What advice would you give a friend who was trying to do the same thing? (Sometimes it's easier to think of solutions for others than for yourself.)
- What *ridiculous* solutions can you include as well as more sensible ones?
- What helpful ideas would others (for example, your family, friends or colleagues at work) suggest?
- What approaches have you tried in the past in similar circumstances?

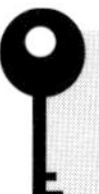

Key point

If you feel stuck, sometimes doing this task with someone you trust can be helpful.

Example: Sam's ideas

Sam has made a list of ideas to help her limit her preparation time to a sensible amount.

- I could pay someone else to do the preparation for me!
- I could get out my lesson plans from last year and use those.
- I could ask my colleagues if any of them have shorter lesson plans I could use.

➜

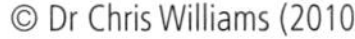

- I could set a limit on the amount of time I spend preparing for any one lesson.
- I could aim to do most of the preparation in the times allocated for that at school.
- I could plan some evenings off so Andrea and I can spend some uninterrupted time together.

Now write down your list (including ridiculous ideas at first) here:

Step 3: Look at the pros and cons of each possible solution

Example: Sam's list of pros and cons

Idea	Pros (advantages)	Cons (disadvantages)
I could pay someone else to do the preparation for me!	It would be no effort for me	I can't afford it. It's a great fantasy though
I could get out my lesson plans from last year and use those	It would be very efficient	There's no real downside. I have them filed away. It would cover 75 per cent of the lessons. Some have changed but not all
I could ask my colleagues if any of them have shorter lesson plans I could use	It would be great if I could get some of the missing 25 per cent of lessons from someone else	It might not help that much because it's hard to give someone else's lesson. It would get me started though
I could set a limit on the amount of time I spend on preparing for any one lesson	I know I need to do that. It's got out of hand	The main worry I'd have is if this means that I mess up the lessons as a result. I'd be very worried if I didn't prepare them enough
I could aim to do most of the preparation in the times allocated for that at school	That's a really good goal to have. At least I'm being paid for that time	I don't know a single teacher who can manage to get all their preparation done then. But I could make sure I use that time as efficiently as possible
I could plan some evenings off so Andrea and I can spend some uninterrupted time together	That would be good – we really need that time. I'm worried if we don't improve things we'll end up splitting up	I'd be worried I might not get everything prepared enough. I don't want to mess up the classes

Write your list of ideas into the following table, along with the pros and cons of each suggestion.

My suggestions from Step 2	Pros (advantages)	Cons (disadvantages)

By doing this task you have made a big effort in trying to stop an unhelpful behaviour. You have recognised your unhelpful behaviour and you are ready to tackle it.

Step 4: Now choose one of the solutions

Now you need to choose a solution that is realistic and you think will be likely to succeed. Choose something that gets you moving in the right direction. It should be small enough to be possible, but big enough to move you forwards. Look at the table you made in Step 3 to help with this.

Example: Sam's choice

Sam realises that she's got some very good ideas there. She feels tempted to try all except the first one. But she remembers that to make effective changes, she needs to move forward slowly and with a clear plan. She therefore decides to start with her second solution: to get out her lesson plans from last year and use those.

Write your choice here:

Now check your choice against some of the **Questions for effective change**:

- Will your chosen solution be useful for changing how you are?

Yes ☐ No ☐

- Is it a specific task so that you will know when you have done it?

Yes ☐ No ☐

- Is it realistic, practical and achievable?

Yes ☐ No ☐

Step 5: Plan the steps needed to carry it out

Write down the practical steps needed to carry out your plan. Try to be very clear in your plan so that you know **what** you are going to do, and **when** you are going to do it.

Try also to think through anything that could block you doing it, and make a plan of how you would tackle any blocks that occur.

Example: Sam gets out her lesson plans from last year

This sounds straightforward, but there's actually quite a lot to do here. I'm glad I only decided to make this one change to start with.

- Firstly, I need to get my files out of the garage. At least I know where they are.
- I then need to make a list of the lessons that we are doing this term.
- After this I need to hook out the lesson plans we are covering this week and next week. I'll need to have my timetable at hand for this.
- I need to pick a day when I've got time to do this and won't be too stressed with what's coming up tomorrow. I think I will start on Friday and Saturday this week.
- I'll use the plans for preparing half the lessons on the first two days of the week. This will take the pressure off me during the rest of the week. I could easily do the rest in my preparation slots at school.

Thinking what might block things:

- I could get side-tracked and start to organise all my old lesson plans. I do have a bad habit of starting one job and then going off at a tangent. To avoid this happening, I'm going to just pick out the folder we used in the same term last year and put the rest straight back into the garage.
- I could start reading through all the lessons – which will take ages. Again, I'm going to have to be very clear and just skim through them and find the ones I need this term, and focus on the ones for the next two weeks.
- I may be tempted to put this off – because I get so anxious thinking about what's coming up. I'm going to find the time though, and ask if Andrea can help me. I'm sure she'll help.

Sam also thinks of a back-up plan in case her first plan doesn't work:

- If for whatever reason I can't get started on Friday then I'll start it on Saturday.

Now write down your plan here:

What if you think that there's something that may block your plan? Write down what you could do to unblock it.

Remember that your plan needs to be a small step that you can achieve. Is it small and slow enough? If not go back and write it down again.

Now check your plan against the rest of the **Questions for effective change**:

Q

- Does your plan make clear what you are going to do and when you are going to do it?

  Yes ☐ No ☐

- Is it an activity that won't be easily blocked or prevented by practical problems?

  Yes ☐ No ☐

- Will it help you to learn useful things even if it doesn't work out perfectly?

  Yes ☐ No ☐

Finally, before you carry on, try to think through what you will do if your initial plan doesn't work out.

Write your back-up plan here:

Step 6: Carry out the plan

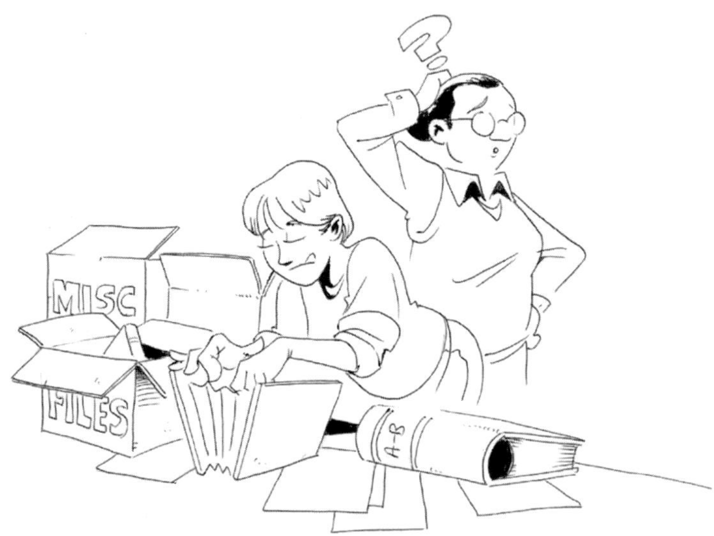

Your task is to carry out this plan during the next week.

Here's where you find out if all that planning has helped you get a good plan.

Pay attention to any thoughts and fears about what will happen before, during and after you have completed your plan. Write any thoughts/fears you noticed here:

Try to do your plan anyway.

Good luck!

Step 7: Review the outcome

Example: Sam's review of her plan

Sam tells Andrea about her plan. Andrea is keen to help and thinks it's a very good idea. That Friday evening they go out into the garage and find 10 boxes of notes. Sam had thought she had written on each box which term it covered, but this wasn't the case. She starts to get flustered and thinks about abandoning her plan. Andrea really helps though by saying there's plenty of time. They start checking through each box in turn and find that the third box they look at is the correct one. They bring it into the kitchen together.

Sam has already put the term's timetable out on the table. She and Andrea quickly look through the box and find the lesson plans for the same time period. Luckily only two of the lessons for next week are different from last year. Although tempted to keep looking, Sam closes up the box and takes out only the lesson plans she needs for the coming two weeks. ➔

She and Andrea then have a nice evening in. On Saturday and Sunday Sam prepares half of the lessons for the first two days of the week, using her old lesson plans. This takes her far less time than she thought it would. Because she has her old plans she feels confident. She starts on Monday and finds things go far better. She is able to keep up with the work more easily. She feels more in control.

Now write down what happened in your plan here:

Q

- Was your plan successful?

  Yes ☐ No ☐

- Did it help improve things?

  Yes ☐ No ☐

- Did any problems arise?

  Yes ☐ No ☐

What have you learned from doing this?

Write down any helpful lessons or information you have learned from what happened. If things didn't go quite as you hoped, try to learn from what happened.

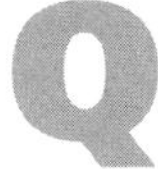
How could you make things different during your next attempt to tackle an unhelpful behaviour?

Were you too ambitious or unrealistic in choosing the target you did?

Planning the next steps

Now that you have reviewed how your first planned target went, the next step is to plan another change to build on this. You will need to slowly build on what you have done in a step-by-step way.

You have the choice to:

- Stop things now. You have achieved what you wanted to.
- Focus on the same problem area some more.
- Choose a new unhelpful behaviour to work on.

There are pros and cons of each of these choices. Think about these, then make your choice.

Next, go on to consider your **short-term**, **medium-term** and **longer-term** targets. This means, where you want to be in a few weeks' time (short term), in a few months' time (medium term) or in a year's time (long term).

Example: Sam's short-term, medium-term and longer-term targets

Sam's **short-term plan** over the next week or so: *I want to keep using my old lesson plans and prepare half the lessons at home in advance – the rest I will do at school.*

Sam's **medium-term plan** over the next few weeks: *I'm going to ask around and see if anyone has taught the topics I haven't done before. If I can borrow their ideas from last year I'll be a lot more efficient.*

Sam's **longer-term plan** over the next few months: *I want to learn some more ways of calming down when things build up.* She decides she is going to learn a relaxation technique, using the Anxiety Control Module available on **www.livinglifetothefull.com**. She gets the free relaxation download and listens to it on her MP3 player. Both she and Andrea get on far better – and slowly things get back to normal at school and at home.

Now it's your turn. In creating your plan:

Do:

- Plan to alter **only** one or two things over the next week.
- Plan to slowly alter things in a step-by-step way.
- Use the **questions for effective change** to check that the next step is always well planned.
- Write down your action plan in detail so that you know exactly what to do this week.

Don't:

- Try to alter too many things all at once.
- Choose something that is too hard a target to start with.
- Be negative and think 'Nothing can be done, it's a waste of time'. Experiment to find out if this negative thinking is actually true.

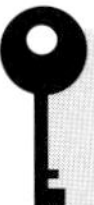

Key point

Remember, hurrying/escaping, trying to feel safe in unhelpful ways, and trying to distract yourself from fears are three main things that can get in the way. These behaviours will damage your attempts to make changes unless you can tackle them. As you make your plans and review your progress, build in checks to make sure you aren't falling into these patterns.

Your short-term, medium-term and longer-term plans

Your short-term plan – what might you do over the next week or so? This is the next step you need to plan.

Your medium-term plan – what might you aim towards doing over the next few weeks – the next few steps?

Your longer-term plan – where do you want to be in a few months or so?

Remember to plan slow, steady changes. This will help you to rebuild your confidence, and increase your control over any unhelpful behaviours.

Summary

In this workbook you have:

- Discovered how some things you do can prevent you tackling anxiety.
- Found out about how some activities can actually make you feel worse.
- Learned some helpful ways to tackle unhelpful behaviours.
- Made a clear plan to reduce an unhelpful behaviour.
- Planned some next steps to build on this.

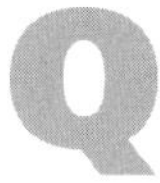

What have I learnt from this workbook?

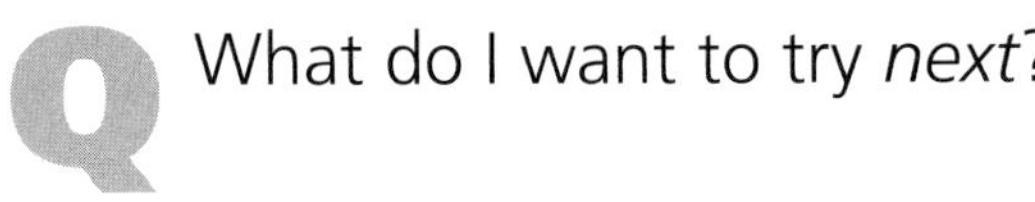

Putting what you have learned into practice

Can we encourage you with this plan? By taking small steps and keeping going large successes can be achieved. Don't try to solve every problem at once. Instead do things at a pace that is right for you. Build changes one step at a time.

Getting more help

The books *The Things You Do That Mess You Up* and *Are You Strong Enough to Keep Your Temper?* have more hints and tips for dealing with unhelpful responses. These books and linked, freely downloadable colour worksheets to help you spot unhelpful actions and work on changing them are available from **www.fiveareas.com**.

My notes

My Unhelpful behaviour diary

Day and date	Morning	Afternoon	Evening
Monday			
Tuesday			
Wednesday			
Thursday			
Friday			
Saturday			
Sunday			

Remember to record every time that you do the unhelpful behaviour. Record **what** you do, and **how long** you do it for. Try to ask **what led to it occurring**, and what the **consequences were** of the behaviour for you and others.

Overcoming Anxiety, Stress and Panic

A Five Areas Approach

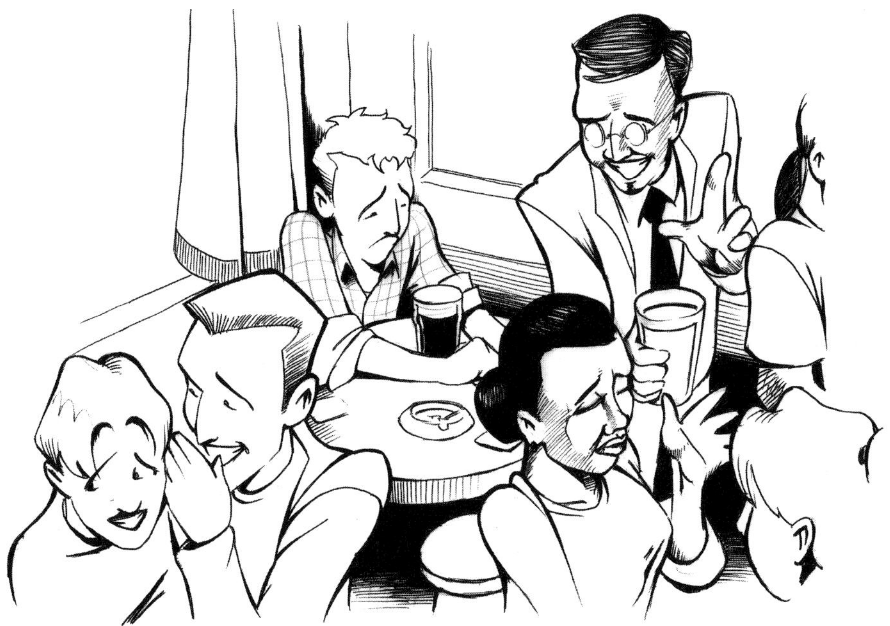

Stress, alcohol and drugs

www.livinglifetothefull.com
www.fiveareas.com

Dr Chris Williams

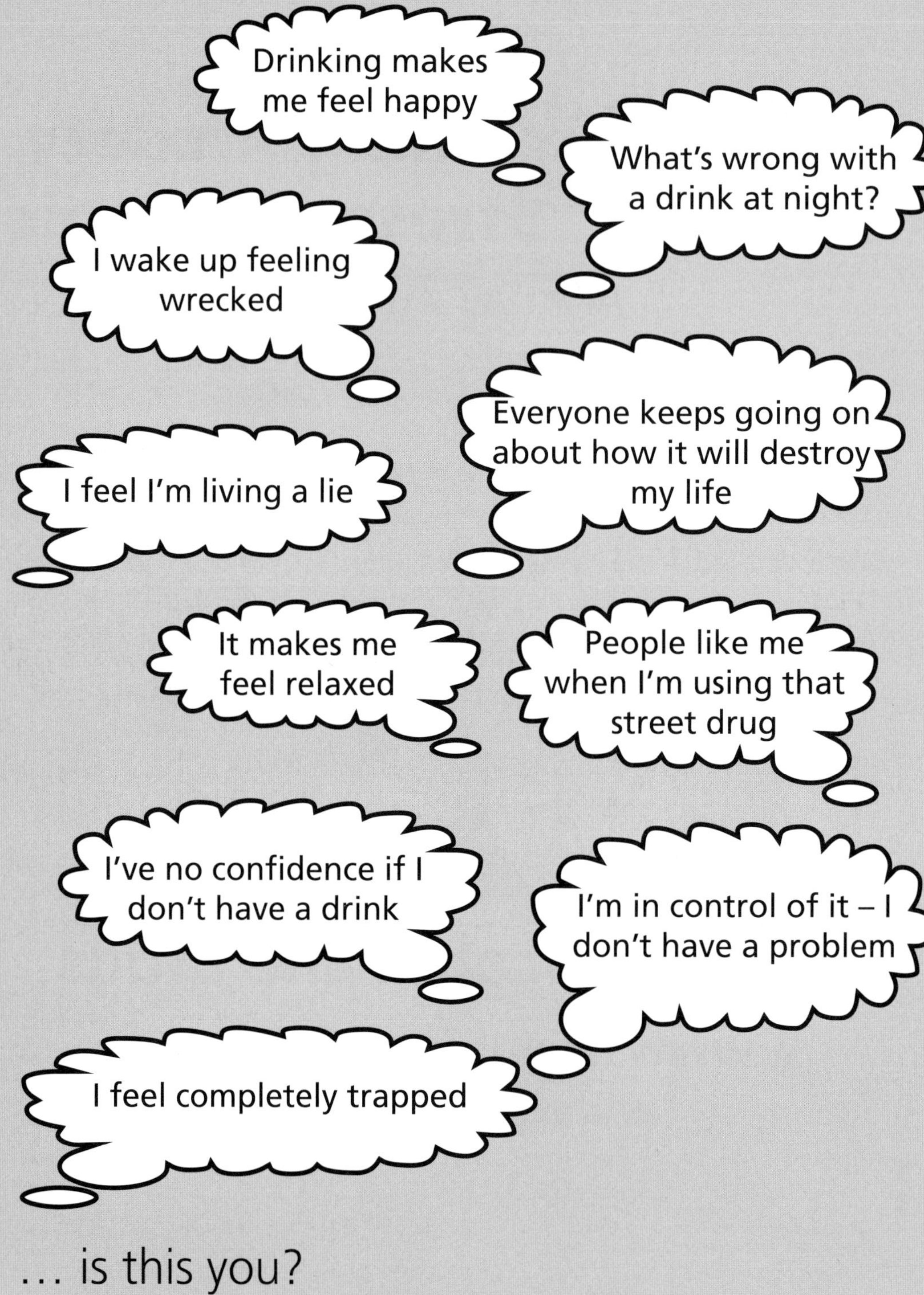
Drinking makes me feel happy
What's wrong with a drink at night?
I wake up feeling wrecked
Everyone keeps going on about how it will destroy my life
I feel I'm living a lie
It makes me feel relaxed
People like me when I'm using that street drug
I've no confidence if I don't have a drink
I'm in control of it – I don't have a problem
I feel completely trapped

… is this you?

If so, … this **workbook is for you**.

If you are misusing alcohol or street drugs you have a serious problem.

In this workbook you will:

- Learn some useful facts about alcohol and street drugs.
- Discover how alcohol and street drugs can make your anxiety and stress worse.
- Work out what effect they're having on you.
- Plan some next steps to bring about change if you have a problem.

Alcohol and street drugs are widely used socially – for fun, for relaxation and for enjoyment. But they can both be misused. Also, buying street drugs is illegal. Importantly, alcohol and street drugs can cause or worsen anxiety.

Using alcohol

Surveys show that many people have drink problems. Alcohol is often part of a night out and spending time with friends. Have you been drinking to:

- Fit in with the crowd?
- Enjoy the effects of drink?
- Block out uncomfortable feelings such as stress?

If you've been drinking a lot of alcohol for weeks or months it can be affecting your mood, your body and your relationships. It can actually make you feel more anxious, irritable or depressed.

This means you get into a vicious circle: the more you drink – the worse you feel – and the worse you feel – the more you drink.

The recommended **highest levels of alcohol for adults** to drink in one week are:

- Women: no more than 2–3 units a day and no more than 14 units a week.
- Men: no more than 3–4 units a day and no more than 21 units a week.

The amounts are less (and sometimes much less) for younger people, depending on your age and weight.

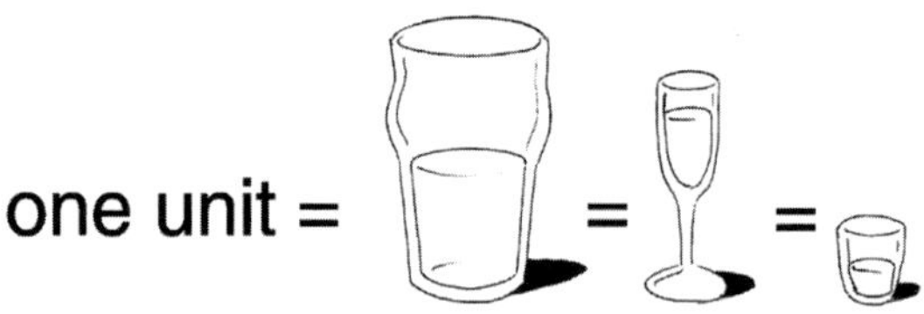

1 unit is = half a pint of bitter or lager – or far less if it is a strong beer, or 1 **small** glass of wine, or one measure of spirits (for example, whisky or gin).

These values vary because stronger lagers or beers, or fortified wines, contain far more than one unit of alcohol.

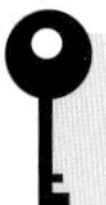

Key point

Always look at the back of the bottle, where you'll find how many units of alcohol there are in standard size glasses for that particular drink. You can also work it out using the online calculator available at www.units.nhs.uk.

Also remember that glass sizes vary in how much they hold.

Using street drugs

People use street drugs for similar reasons to drinking alcohol. There are lots of different street drugs. And even when you think you may be buying one type on the street, it may be contaminated with all sorts of other drugs. Some drugs are known to cause anxiety and panic, for example cocaine and amphetamines. Anxiety can therefore be worsened by using these drugs.

Different drugs have different effects, but there are some effects which are common to all drugs and alcohol.

For more information about street drugs, visit the Talk to Frank website (**www.talktofrank.com**).

Recording what you drink and what drugs you use

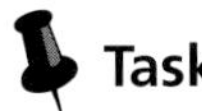 **Task**

Everybody is different. Whether you are drinking or taking street drugs, a **good first step** is to record how much you use. Remember that most people tend to think they have a lot less than they actually have.

Q How many units of alcohol do you drink?

In one day:

- What drink? _________
- How much? _________
- How many times? _________

In one week:

- What drink? _________
- How much? _________
- How many times? _________

How many units is that per week? ___ units

How much are you spending a week on drink? £_________

Q What street drugs are you taking?

In one day:

- What drug? _________
- How much? _________
- How many times? _________

In one week:

- What drug? _________
- How much? _________
- How many times? _________

How much are you spending per week on drugs? £_________

The best way of finding out how much you drink or use in a week is to keep a **diary**. You'll find one at the back of this workbook (page 225). Try to **record each and every time** you drink alcohol or use drugs. At the end of the week, add up the amount you have taken.

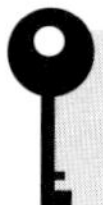

Key point

Remember to record everything you drink/take. If you are drinking/using drugs on a regular basis and/or at a high dose, it may prevent you getting better. Record some brief notes about the consequences (positive and negative) for you and others of each time you drink or take street drugs.

How alcohol and drugs affect you

When you drink a large amount of alcohol or take a large dose of drugs – or regularly drink or take drugs at low doses – they can cause several problems. Some of these are described below.

Thinking/psychological changes

People often drink or use drugs to improve how they feel. But actually these things can cause you to feel more anxious or depressed. They also prevent your anxiety or depression getting better.

Drinking and taking drugs can:

- Worsen worry and cause panic attacks.
- Lead to sudden bouts of confusion or violence.
- Damage your concentration and memory, so that you find it hard to learn and remember new information.
- Worsen your ability to fall asleep and to have a refreshing night's sleep.
- Cause you to become fearful, and increasingly suspicious and mistrustful of others.
- Lead to addiction with craving if you stop taking them abruptly.

Drinking and taking drugs can also make you feel irritable. Your personality changes, but in such a subtle way that you don't realise that you're changing as a result of your habit. You may become withdrawn and stop taking interest in other people or the things around you.

People can occasionally develop severe mental health disorders, which can continue in the long term. For example, having hallucinations (seeing or hearing things that aren't there) or delusions (believing something is true when it clearly isn't). These illnesses can be terrifying to have and cause high levels of anxiety.

Q Do you have any of the mental health symptoms described above?

(Note: You may need to ask people around you.)

Yes ☐ No ☐ Sometimes ☐

Physical changes

- The most common symptom of drinking too much is having a hangover. This includes feeling sick, having headaches and becoming dehydrated (this is when your body doesn't have the amount of water it needs to function properly).
- Both alcohol and drugs can lead to addiction. If you take a lot of alcohol or drugs, you can become dependent on them (alcohol/drug dependency). You can also become dependent on the so-called 'soft' drugs, for example cannabis – some types of which are not 'soft' in effect at all.
- If someone drinks or uses drugs at a high level for some time and then suddenly stops them they get **withdrawal symptoms** such as sweatiness and feeling sick. Withdrawal is a serious medical condition. Symptoms of mild withdrawal include anxiety, tension and sleeplessness. More severe withdrawal causes confusion, agitation and hallucinations. The person may even go into a coma, or have fits/seizures or wet themselves.
- Alcohol can cause damage to parts of your body. For example it can cause stomach ulcers (holes in the lining of your stomach) and can damage your liver. It can also damage your brain so that you start having epileptic fits. Other important body organs such as the pancreas can also be damaged, causing you extreme pain.
- Taking drugs can reduce your ability to fight off infections or serious disease.
- Drugs can also cause **lung cancer** and heart problems, or you can have a stroke. You can also start having fits or your body temperature regulation can get upset. Drugs can also cause you to get suddenly confused. People can even die suddenly as drugs can be toxic to many body organs.

Q Do you have any of the physical symptoms described above?

Yes ☐ No ☐ Sometimes ☐

If you answered 'Yes' or 'Sometimes', then it is important that you ask your doctor for advice about what to do next.

Social changes

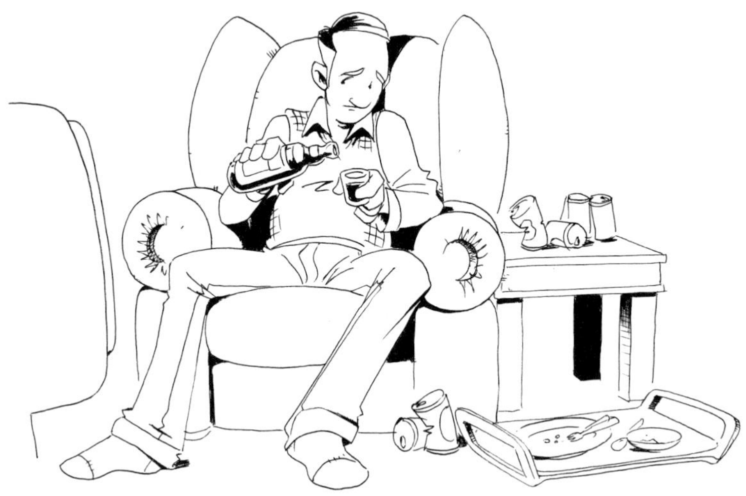

- You may have problems at home such as **arguments** with family and friends. You may feel snappier and more irritable than usual.
- You may get into **debt**.
- You may struggle to keep up with your work – or with the house. You may ignore or neglect people around you such as your partner, children or friends.
- **Accidents and violence** are also common social consequences of alcohol dependency.

You have reduced motivation and energy, so that everything apart from drinking seems too much an effort. You may stop going out and just stay at home, drinking alone.

Q Do you have any of the social changes described above?

Yes ☐ No ☐ Sometimes ☐

Q Based on your answers to all the questions above, overall, do you think that you have drink/drug problems?

Yes ☐ No ☐ Sometimes ☐

If you have answered 'Yes' or 'Sometimes' to this question, this is an alert that you need to make some changes.

Key point

Drinking or using drugs in ways that can harm you or others is likely to cause you increasing problems in each of the areas described above. **You need to tackle your problem now.**

Don't be tempted to downplay or ignore things and believe it isn't a problem. **Ignoring things is often part of the problem.**

How your drinking affects you

The good news is that if this applies to you, you can make changes.

Example: Andrea's drinking

Andrea has started to drink more to try to cope with symptoms of stress. Her drinking is now affecting both her and her partner Sam.

However, Andrea doesn't recognise she has a drink problem. Instead she sees drink as something that is helpful. This is because she hasn't worked out the unhelpful effects of the drinking on her life. She needs to start looking at the downsides of her drinking as well as the immediate benefits. This means looking at the short-term and longer-term effects of her daily drinking on herself, and her partner. ➜

How is Andrea's drinking affecting her?

In the short term:

- **Physically**: Andrea is noticing she feels shaky if she doesn't have a drink every day.
- **Psychologically**: She feels it makes her more relaxed and helps her sleep at night to begin with. But then she wakes up and has to go to the toilet. So she feels too tired to get up in the morning and sleeps in to catch up on sleep. This worsens her sleeping pattern. She also feels far worse in the morning when she's been drinking more the night before. She notices that unless she drinks each night she feels twitchy and stressed and can't get off to sleep at all.
- **Socially**: Andrea's partner Sam is worried about her. They keep having arguments about this. Andrea is worried that it's affecting their relationship.

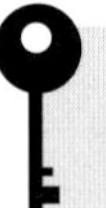

Key point

Both *helpful* and *unhelpful* behaviours make us feel better in the short term. But in the longer term, our unhelpful behaviours such as heavy drinking backfire. They worsen how we or others feel. They become part of our problem.

The good news is that if this applies to you, you can make changes.

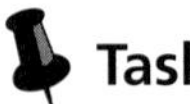

Task

Now think about your own drink or drug use or both.

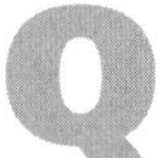

How does my drinking or drug use affect me and the people around me in the short term?

- Physically:

- Psychologically (especially how does it affect any anxious feelings or depression):

- Socially (on you and others, for example, your family, children, friends):

Q How has my drinking or drug use affected me and the people around me in the longer term? (Look back over the past six to 12 months.)

- Physically:

- Psychologically (especially how does it affect any anxious feelings or depression):

- Socially (on you and others):

If after reading this workbook you have discovered that your drinking or drug use is causing harm to you or others, then **you need to tackle it**.

Q What have I learnt from this workbook?

Q What do I want to try *next*?

How to make changes

Try to reduce your overall intake of alcohol or drugs each week:

- Do this slowly in steady steps over several weeks.
- If possible, plan to eventually have **at least two days** each week without any drink or drugs to allow your body to recover.

Discuss your goals and how to achieve this with your doctor.

If you're drinking or using street drugs at a far higher level

If you stop drinking or taking the drugs too quickly, you may notice some symptoms of withdrawal. This is probably the reason why so many people don't manage to tackle this problem. But it's still possible to make changes – and it's even more important to do so if you're having a lot of drinks or drugs.

To change yourself successfully you need to cut down the amount you're taking in a **slow, step-by-step manner**. You may find the *Things you do that worsen your anxiety (unhelpful behaviours)* workbook useful for some ideas of how to plan this, so that it moves you in the right direction.

If you're taking drugs or drinking alcohol at higher levels, it's best to make these changes together with some closer help and advice from your GP, health visitor, local drug or alcohol support services or other healthcare practitioner.

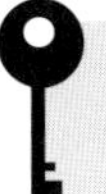

Key point

If you regularly use street drugs, or drink a lot of alcohol, you should discuss this with someone who can help.

Extra resources

Look at your local *Yellow Pages*, and also the following national organisations:

1. **NHS Direct (England and Wales).** NHS Direct will help and advise on any aspect of drug and alcohol use (tel: **0845 46 47**; **www.nhsdirect.nhs.uk**).
2. **NHS24 (Scotland)**. If you live in Scotland ring NHS24 for advice and assessment (tel: **0845 24 24 24**; **www.nhs24.com**).
3. **Royal College of Psychiatrists**. The College has an information sheet about drugs and alcohol. You can get this from their website (**www.rcpsych.ac.uk**).
4. **Talk to Frank**. This website has stories, information and resources about drugs. It also has information for family and friends. You can talk on the phone and ask for information from a counsellor. Or you can email or access help online (tel: **0800 776 600**; **www.talktofrank.com**). Please note that Frank is **not** a real person but the website is a way for you to get advice and information about drugs.

5. Alcohol Focus Scotland (**www.alcohol-focus-scotland.org.uk**), NHS Choices – Alcohol: know your limits (**www.units.nhs.uk**) and Drinkaware (**www.drinkaware.co.uk**) are three other useful websites.

Summary

In this workbook you have learnt:

- Some useful facts about alcohol and street drugs.
- How alcohol and street drugs can affect you and your family and make anxiety and stress worse.
- How you can work out what effects they're having on you.
- How to plan some next steps to bring about change if you have a problem.

My notes

Drink/street drug diary: my week

Day and date	Morning	Afternoon	Evening	Total units or cost
Monday				Total units/amount per day = Cost/day £ =
Tuesday				Total units/amount per day = Cost/day £ =
Wednesday				Total units/amount per day = Cost/day £ =
Thursday				Total units/amount per day = Cost/day £ =
Friday				Total units/amount per day = Cost/day £ =
Saturday				Total units/amount per day = Cost/day £ =
Sunday				Total units/amount per day = Cost/day £ =
Weekly total				**Units =** **Cost =**

Overcoming Anxiety, Stress and Panic
A Five Areas Approach

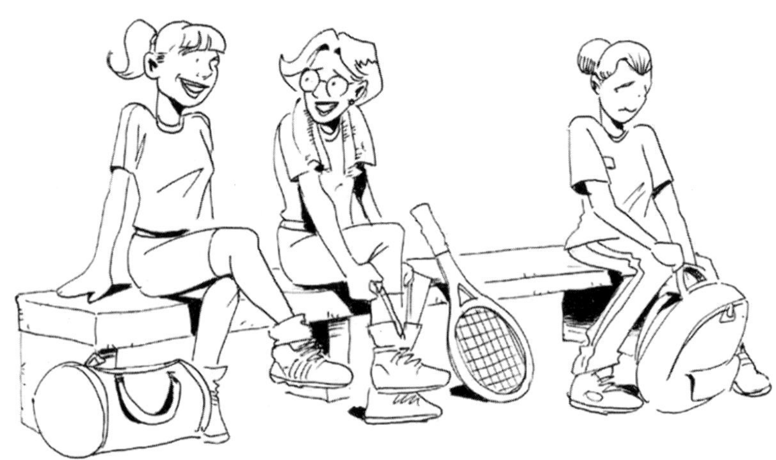

Facing fears and overcoming avoidance

www.livinglifetothefull.com
www.fiveareas.com

Dr Chris Williams

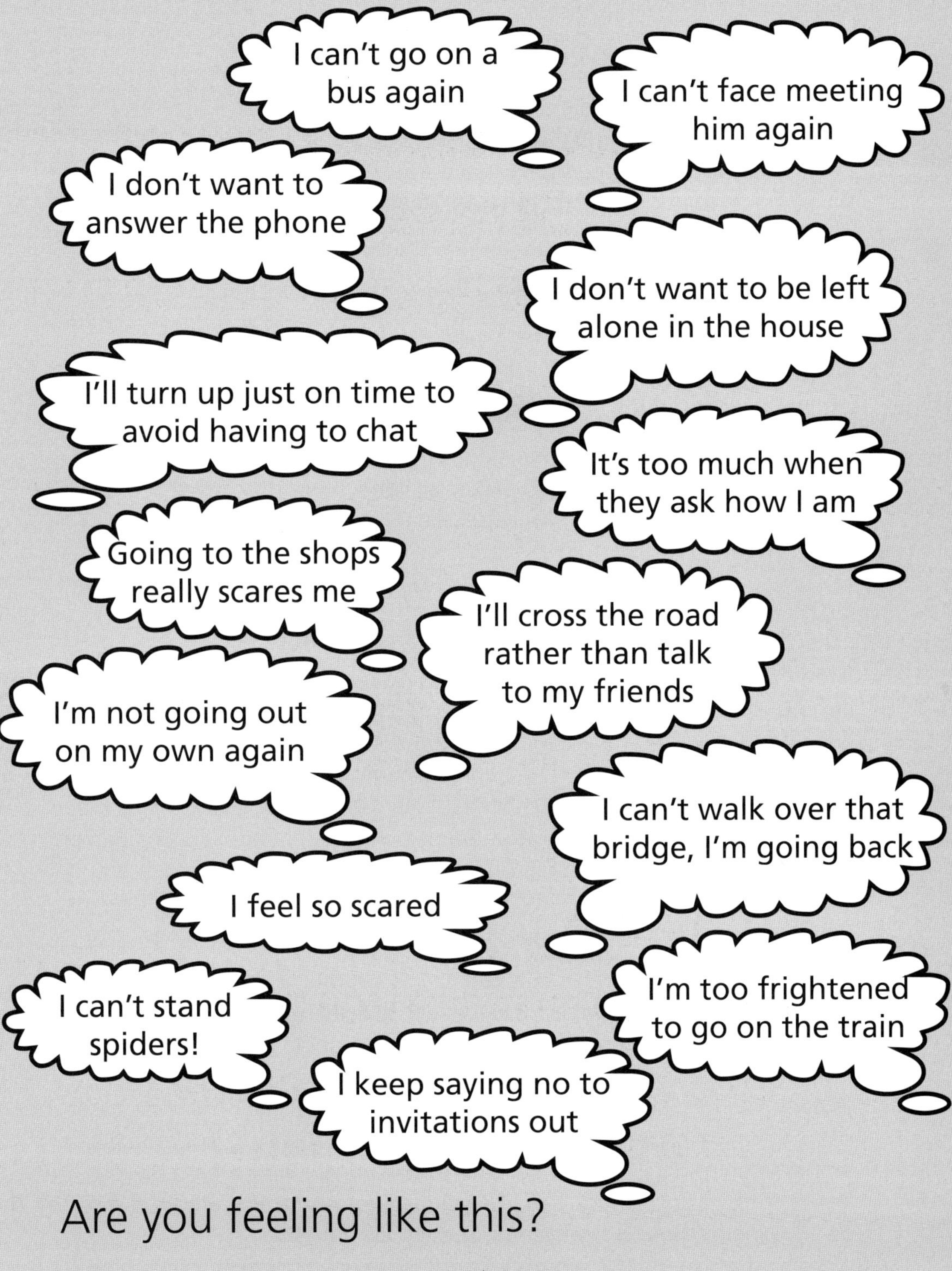
I can't go on a bus again
I can't face meeting him again
I don't want to answer the phone
I don't want to be left alone in the house
I'll turn up just on time to avoid having to chat
It's too much when they ask how I am
Going to the shops really scares me
I'll cross the road rather than talk to my friends
I'm not going out on my own again
I can't walk over that bridge, I'm going back
I feel so scared
I can't stand spiders!
I'm too frightened to go on the train
I keep saying no to invitations out

Are you feeling like this?

If so, … this **workbook is for you**.

In this workbook you will:

- Find out why you feel like avoiding things that seem scary.
- Learn how avoiding things can make you feel worse.
- Decide on a clear plan to make slow, steady changes to tackle avoidance.
- Plan some next steps to build on this.

How worrying fears affect how you feel

Have you been worrying about things and feeling you can't cope? Or do you feel that things will go wrong? Sometimes these fears can keep building up. If your anxiety reaches a very high level (panic), you may want to leave or escape from the situation that's making you feel like this.

Here's how panic and high levels of anxiety can affect you in five key areas of your life:

- **Area 1: People and events around you**. Sometimes people can become anxious about being in particular situations or places. For example, you may be anxious about having a one-to-one conversation, or about how you behave in a group. You may find new challenges can seem scary. For example, starting a new job for the first time. There are so many things that can make you feel anxious. Phobias are particular fears that build up and up, for example the fear of going into busy shops, or getting on a bus, or the fear of heights or spiders. During a panic attack, or if you have a phobia, just thinking about being in that situation can cause fear, and you can get into patterns of avoiding these situations.
- **Area 2: Your thinking**. When you are feeling a little anxious you tend to have worrying thoughts about the past or what's going on now. Or you may have concerns about the future. Sometimes when you are extremely anxious, you may become very scared – predicting that the very worst, most awful thing will happen. This is called 'catastrophic thinking'. For example, during a panic attack you can become convinced *you will collapse, have a heart attack, suffocate, collapse, die, go mad, lose control, wet yourself or do anything else that is humiliating*. These scary thoughts can make you feel worse and worse. All this worry can turn you in on yourself and cause you to avoid situations that seem stressful or scary. They affect how you feel and also what you do.

- **Area 3: Your feelings (emotions)**. When you are worried just a little, you feel anxious and stressed but you can cope with it. But if you begin to feel very scared, you can become panicky and terrified that the very worst will happen. Sometimes you can feel all sorts of other emotions. For example, you may feel irritable and angry at things you would usually cope with or guilty if you have let people down.
- **Area 4: Altered physical symptoms**. When you feel scared your body also reacts. When you are feeling just a little anxious, you may notice feelings of tension, or you may feel fidgety or find it hard to get off to sleep. When you are feeling even more anxious, you are likely to notice stronger physical symptoms. You may feel hot, sweaty, shaky or cold, your heart rate goes up and you take rapid shallow breaths, and you may feel dizzy or faint. You may also have an urge to go to the toilet or feel sick. All of these are common symptoms that can happen to anyone at times of anxiety.

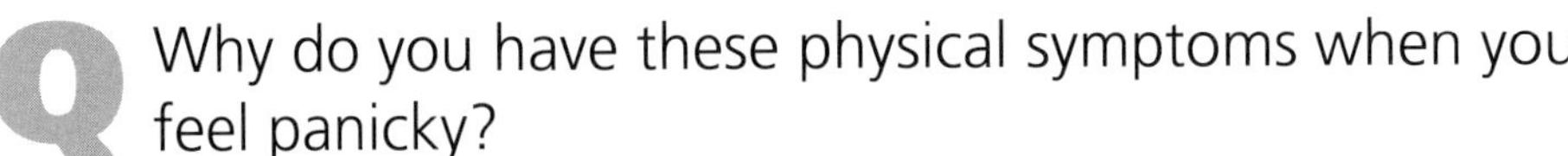

Why do you have these physical symptoms when you feel panicky?

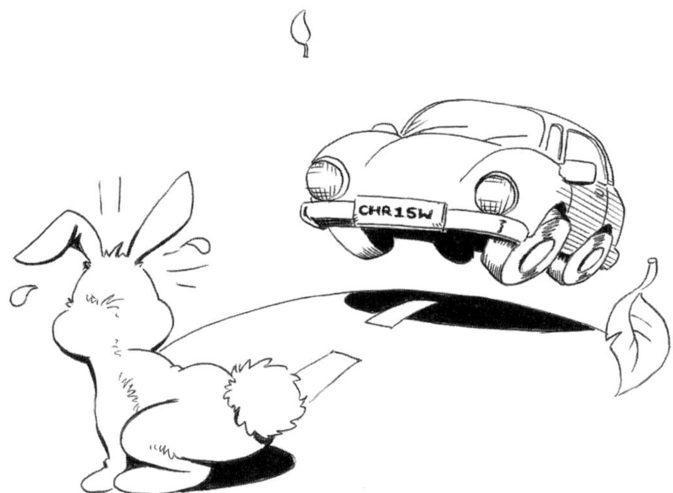

Your body reacts to frightening thoughts just as it would to a physical danger. The **fight or flight adrenaline response** creates all of the symptoms described above. Your heart rate and breathing both speed up so that your muscles are ready to react to defend yourself or run away. This is very useful when the danger is real, but not when it is caused just by scary thoughts.

You can find out more about these sorts of symptoms and the fight or flight adrenaline response in the *Understanding panic and phobias* workbook.

- **Area 5: Altered behaviour or activity levels**. The current workbook you are reading focuses on one of the most common things that people do when they feel anxious – avoiding things as a result of anxious fears.

Avoidance and its effect on you

Some of the things people start avoiding when they feel anxious or scared are:

- **Going to particular places or situations** where you think you will feel worse. For example, someone who is very nervous about talking to others will try hard to avoid situations such as going to a back-to-work group, a church, synagogue or temple group, or a parent and toddler meeting. Or they **may go but try to arrive late** and then leave early – or avoid talking to people there. People who get panicky or have a phobia will go to great lengths to avoid situations where they might face their fear. So, people who fear feeling worse in shops (sometimes called agoraphobia) will avoid going into larger, busier shops. Similarly someone who is terrified of falling from a height or of being stung by a wasp will try hard to avoid these situations. Does that sound like you?
- **Activities you are scared of**. You may look to others to help you with particular tasks or decisions. For example, some mothers worry about bathing their baby in case they drop or hurt them. Or you may avoid doing things that seem scary, for example travelling somewhere, going for an interview, dancing in public or talking to someone at a meal.
- **Your physical health**. Sometimes you may have worries about how your activities are affecting your physical health. This is sensible if there is a clear reason to limit things – for example, you may have had an operation or you have a condition such as asthma. But sometimes people overdo it. For example, someone with exercise-induced asthma may become so anxious about another attack that they avoid **any** activity. They lose confidence in their ability to do most things 'just in case' it makes them feel worse.

Physical symptoms aren't all caused by feeling low or anxious. If you notice new or worsening physical symptoms, you should see your doctor. But it's worth knowing that anxiety can often raise fears about your physical health, and to think about whether this may be affecting you.

Whatever the cause, when you try to avoid things it adds to your problems by sapping your confidence. Over time, avoidance tends to affect more and more things. That's why it's important to stop it taking over your life.

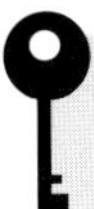

Key point

The problem with avoidance is that it teaches you that the **only** way to deal with a difficult situation is by avoiding it. This worsens your anxiety and saps your confidence. In fact often the best way of tackling your fears is to face them in a planned way. This also helps you test out whether your fears are actually true.

Things I avoid doing

Ask yourself 'What have I stopped or avoided doing because of my worries?'. Remember that at times the avoidance can be quite **subtle**. For example, choosing to go to the shops at a time you know they are quiet, and then rushing through the shopping as quickly as possible.

Write down any examples of avoidance you may have noticed:

Now answer the following questions:

Q Are you avoiding things because they feel too difficult or scary?

Yes ☐ No ☐ Sometimes ☐

Q Has this reduced your confidence in things and led to a more restricted lifestyle?

Yes ☐ No ☐ Sometimes ☐

Q Overall has this worsened how you feel?

Yes ☐ No ☐ Sometimes ☐

If you have answered 'Yes' or 'Sometimes' to all three questions, then avoidance is causing problems for you.

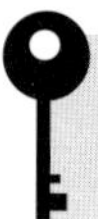

Key point

The good news is that once you have noticed that you are avoiding things, you can begin to start tackling it.

Seven steps to tackling avoidance

You may have tried to stop avoiding things before. But unless you have a clear plan and stick to it, change will be hard to make. Making one change at a time is the key thing to help you move forwards. This may mean choosing at first **not** to focus on other areas.

By setting targets you can focus on how to make the changes needed to get better. To do this, you need to decide your:

- **Short-term** targets – these are the changes you can make today, tomorrow and the next week.
- **Medium-term** targets – these are the changes to be put in place over the next few weeks.
- **Long-term** targets – this is where you want to be in six months or a year.

By working through the seven steps below you can learn how to plan clear ways of overcoming avoidance. The aim is to slowly plan **specific** activities to boost your confidence and tackle avoidance. The good news is that you plan this one step at a time. And you can keep practising a step until you feel comfortable at that step. That way it never seems too much or too scary.

Step 1: Identify and clearly define your problem

The following table lists the activities that people commonly avoid when they are anxious or panicky. You will probably have noticed avoiding at least some of these activities.

Checklist: Identifying your patterns of worsening avoidance

As a result of how you feel, are you:	Tick here if you have noticed this – even if just sometimes
Avoiding specific situations, objects or places because of fears about what harm might result? For example, shops, heights, spiders, wasps or butterflies	☐
Avoiding specific activities such as dancing, presenting or performing in front of others	☐
Putting off dealing with important practical problems (both large and small)? For example, delaying paying a bill when money is tight	☐
Avoiding being with others in crowded or hot places, or busy and large shops?	☐
Not really being honest with others? For example, saying *yes* when you really mean *no* or by not saying things that you really want to	☐
Trying hard to avoid situations that bring about upsetting thoughts/memories?	☐
Avoiding opening or replying to letters?	☐
Sleeping in to avoid doing things or meeting people?	☐
Looking to others to sort things out for you?	☐
Avoiding answering the phone, or the door when people visit?	☐
Avoiding having sex because of anxiety?	☐
Avoiding going on buses, in cars, taxis, etc., or any places where it's hard to escape?	☐
Avoiding being in situations where you may need to talk/do things with others? For example, meeting people or groups of people	☐
Avoiding walking alone far from home?	☐
Stopping attending religious services, night classes or local pubs/clubs because it feels just too much to cope with at present?	☐

Write down any other activities you are avoiding here:

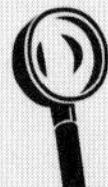

Example: Paul's avoidance

Paul has been invited to join a back-to-work course that starts in four weeks. He feels very anxious about going and fears he will go red and start stuttering. Although he knows he needs to go to the course to help him rebuild his confidence he's feeling hesitant about it.

Choosing a first target

Use the list above to choose a single target that you will focus on to start with. This is particularly important if you have ticked several boxes in the checklist. It isn't possible to work on all these areas at once. Instead you need to decide which **one** area to focus on to start with.

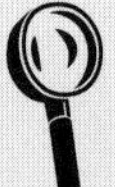

Example: Paul breaks his target into smaller steps

Paul wants to attend the back-to-work course. This starts in four weeks' time. Paul decides he needs to start building his confidence up towards getting there. He has realised that he tries to avoid talking to people, even to the extent of crossing the road if he sees someone ahead he knows.

➔

Paul therefore decides to focus on something that would be a good first step towards getting to the course – building confidence when he's talking to others. This is something that would help tackle a big problem for him, which is affecting whether he can go on the course.

Paul's target: I'm going to focus on feeling more comfortable talking to others.

Write down one problem you want to work on here. (Remember that this should be a problem of avoidance.)

Be a detective

The next thing is to do some research on your avoidance. First, record in detail every time you avoid your chosen problem over several days. At the back of the workbook in the My notes section write down:

- What you avoid.
- When you avoid it.
- How much you do it (for example, don't go out, don't go to the shops, don't say hello – because of worries).
- How long it lasts for.

Try to understand more about your avoidance and why you tend to do it. Work out why you avoid or escape from things at that time, such as:

- The time of day.
- Whether you slept well the night before.
- Who you were with and how they responded.
- How you felt emotionally.
- What went through your mind – what were your fears?

- How you felt emotionally and physically at the time.
- Any other things you did to try to cope or escape.

... and anything else that seems to help explain your reaction.

Write any important things you have learned here:

Check point: is your target a realistic target? Answer the **Questions for change** to find out:

Is your target:

- Clear and realistic and something that you can tackle over the next week or two?

  Yes ☐ No ☐

- Not so scary that you can't face doing it?

  Yes ☐ No ☐

- Still helping you move forwards?

  Yes ☐ No ☐

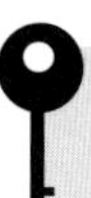

Key point

Sometimes you need to make sure that your first target really is a small, focused problem so that you can tackle it in one step.

Now use your notes to decide if you need to break down your avoidance behaviour into smaller steps that you can target one at a time.

Q Do you need to break the avoidance down into a number of smaller, more achievable targets?

Yes ☐ No ☐

If you answered 'No', then please go straight to Step 2. If you answered 'Yes', then keep reading. Take the target and break it down into smaller steps. Make sure you've chosen a realistic first target and write it here again.

My clear first step is:

Step 2: Think up as many solutions as possible to achieve your initial target

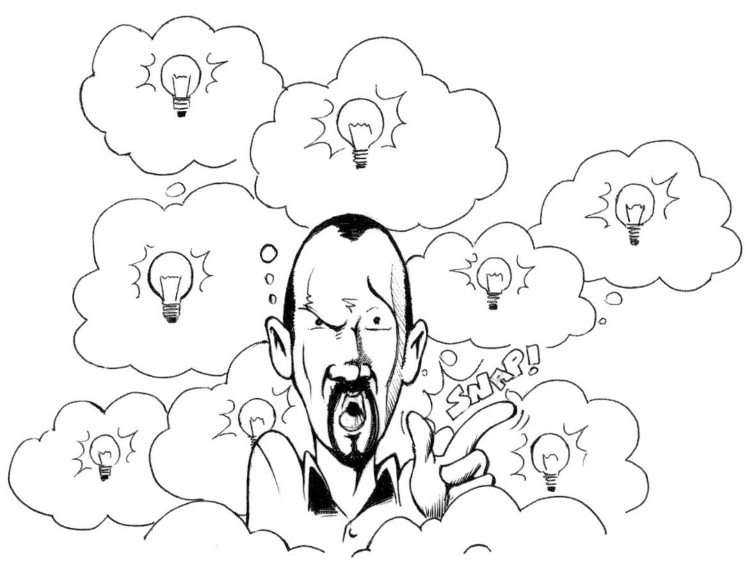

Try to come up with as many ideas as possible. Include completely whacky ideas in your list as well, even if you wouldn't choose to do them. This will help you to **think broadly**. Here are some useful questions to help you to think up possible solutions:

- What advice would you give a friend who was trying to tackle the same problem?
- What ridiculous solutions can you include as well as more sensible ones?
- What helpful suggestions would others make?
- How could you look at the solutions facing you differently? What would you have said before you felt like this, or what might you say about the situation, say in five years' time?
- What approaches have you tried in the past in similar circumstances?

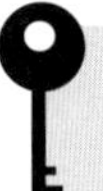

Key point

If you feel stuck, sometimes doing this task with someone you trust can help.

Example: Paul's ideas to help him feel more comfortable talking to others

I could:

- Pay an actor to be my friend and talk to me. I'd feel in charge then!
- Start small – and build up my confidence on the phone.
- Ask a friend to come round to chat so that I can practise talking again with someone who I know likes me.
- Start going again to the photography club I used to attend.

Now write down as many possible options (including ridiculous ideas at first) for your own situation:

Step 3: Look at the pros and cons of each possible solution

Example: Paul's list of pros and cons

Idea	Pros (advantages)	Cons (disadvantages)
Pay an actor to be my friend and talk to me. I'd feel in charge then!	They'd be there all day. I could ask them to be friendly and nice	That's a crazy idea. But wouldn't it be great to to have that much money!
Start small – and build up my confidence on the phone	This is a small step which is great	I'm actually okay on the phone. It's more when I actually am with someone that I start to go red and clam up
Ask a friend to come round to chat so that I can practise talking again with someone who I know likes me	That sounds perfect. If it's someone I trust it wouldn't matter to me as much as someone who's not a friend. I could do that and I think it would help me build my confidence again	I might clam up. But then I don't think that should happen. I just need to plan a few conversation starters for if things go quiet. I think that's okay
Start going again to the photography club I used to attend	Wouldn't that be great! I could go in and suddenly be confident all over again with people I know	It just doesn't seem that realistic. It's too big a step. I'd turn up and just sit alone in the corner feeling embarrassed. Or I'd leave and never go back

Write your own list of ideas into the following table, along with the pros and cons of each suggestion.

My suggestions from Step 2	Pros (advantages)	Cons (disadvantages)

Step 4: Now choose one of the solutions

Choose a solution that is a small step in the right direction and you think will be likely to succeed. Look at the list you made in Step 3 to help you with this.

The best way to tackle avoidance is to plan **steady, slow changes**. In this way, you can rebuild your confidence. The step should be small enough to be possible, but big enough to move you forwards.

Example: Paul's choice

Paul decides to ask his friend Raj to come round to chat, so that he can practise talking again with someone he knows he gets on with.

Key point

The first step you decide on should be something that helps you tackle your avoidance. If it seems scary, it shouldn't be so scary that you can't do it. You must be realistic in your choice so that the target doesn't appear impossible to do.

Write your choice here:

Now check your choice against some of the **Questions for effective change**.

Q Will your chosen step be useful for changing how you are?

Yes ☐ No ☐

Q Is it a specific task so that you will know when you've done it?

Yes ☐ No ☐

Q Is it realistic, practical and achievable?

Yes ☐ No ☐

If you answered 'Yes' to all three questions your chosen step should help start you off. If not, go back to your plan and re-write it so you can answer 'Yes' to each question.

Step 5: Plan the steps needed to carry it out

You need to have a clear plan that will help you to decide exactly **what** you are going to do and **when** you are going to do it. **Write down** the steps needed to carry out your plan. This will help you to think what to do and also think of the possible problems that might arise. An important part of the plan is to try to think what could block the plan from happening or make it hard for you to follow it. That way you can think about how you would respond to keep your plan on track.

Example: Paul's plan

Paul phones his friend Raj, whom he knows from way back at school. They have stayed in close touch since and remain good friends. Raj knows Paul has struggled with depression. But Paul hasn't seen Raj for a few weeks and is a little nervous about how things will go. He therefore decides the following plan: 'Raj will come by at 3 o'clock tomorrow. We can have a cup of tea or coffee and have a chat. If it's good weather we could walk and talk.'

Paul also tries to think of what might go wrong or cause problems. He thinks he may feel uncomfortable about silences. Therefore he plans to make sure he has a few questions to use to get things going if needed. He looks through the hints and tips for starting and keeping conversations going in the *How to ask for what you really need (being assertive)* workbook. He now feels confident Raj and he will have enough things to talk about.

Now write down your plan here:

What if you think that there's something that may block your plan? Write down what you could do next to unblock it.

Now check your plan against the rest of the **Questions for effective change**:

Q Does your plan make clear what you are going to do and when you are going to do it?

Yes ☐ No ☐

Q Is it an activity that won't be easily blocked or prevented by practical problems?

Yes ☐ No ☐

Q Will it help you to learn useful things even if it doesn't work out perfectly?

Yes ☐ No ☐

Step 6: Carry out the plan

Your task now is to carry out your plan during the next week.

As you get ready to put your plan into action be aware of worrying thoughts or fears. One of the best ways of checking how true unhelpful fears are is to act against them and see what happens.

Pay attention to any thoughts and fears you may have about what will happen before, during and after you have completed your plan. Write any thoughts/fears you noticed here:

If things seem just too scary, decide that you will carry out the plan *anyway* and see what happens. If things do seem too scary, then go back to Step 2 (your brainstorm) and pick something that is a less scary first step.

Good luck!

Step 7: Review the outcome

Example: Paul's review

Raj is a little late which makes Paul feel slightly more nervous. He starts making the tea to keep busy. When Raj arrives, Paul is no longer that anxious and they start chatting straight away.

Later, Paul thinks that Raj's visit helped a lot. He also thinks that when he finally gets to the course, he should remember that doing something while waiting helps. Paul really enjoyed the chat with Raj.

Well done on carrying out your plan. Now write down your own review here:

Q Was your plan successful?

Yes ☐ No ☐

Q Did it help improve things?

Yes ☐ No ☐

Q Did any problems arise?

Yes ☐ No ☐

Things that can de-rail your plans

When you feel anxious, there are three common behaviours that can act to keep you feeling anxious and stop you improving.

As a result of how you feel, do you:	Tick here if you have noticed this – even if just sometimes
1. Hurry through your plan and try to leave/escape quickly For example: walking or talking faster, cutting things short, making your excuses and leaving, or even lying that you need to be elsewhere or feel ill	☐
2. Do things that make you feel safer in the short term For example: seeking constant reassurance from others; looking to others to make decisions for you, do things for you, or come along with you when you feel scared; or misusing medication, drink or street drugs to give you false courage and block how you feel	☐
3. Try hard to distract yourself from fearful or worrying thoughts or physical symptoms For example: trying to say positive comments again and again ('I'll be alright, I'll be alright'); trying to think hard of something else (such as counting the tiles on a wall); doing something physical to hurt or distract you from fears (such as clenching your fists, biting your lip, digging your nails into your hand)	☐

Each of the above behaviours seems very attractive at the time. However, they are all ways of subtle avoidance. They make you feelbetter – at the time. But in the long term they can actually worsen how you feel.

If you have noticed that your plan hasn't gone as well as you hoped, check if any of the three behaviours above have de-railed you. If so, you need to take what happened into account when you plan the next step.

What have you learned from doing this?

Write down any helpful lessons or information you have learned from what happened. If things didn't go quite as you hoped, try to learn from what happened.

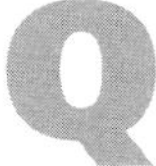

How could you make things different during your next attempt to tackle your avoidance?

Were you too ambitious in choosing the target you did?

Planning the next steps

Now that you have reviewed how your first planned target went, the next step is to plan another change to build on this. You will need to slowly build on what you have done in a step-by-step way.

You have the choice to:

- Stick with the target you have achieved.
- Focus on the same problem area and plan to keep working on this.
- Choose a new area to work on.

There are pros and cons of each of these choices. Think about these when you make your choice.

When you are making this decision, bear in mind that by practising the same step **again and again** over the next few weeks your confidence will grow. Your anxious fears will also get less and last for a shorter and shorter time.

This happens no matter what fear you try to tackle. Facing up to a fear causes it to slowly lose its effect on you. Look at how Paul's fear has reduced.

First time Paul has a friend round: Tuesday at 3pm.

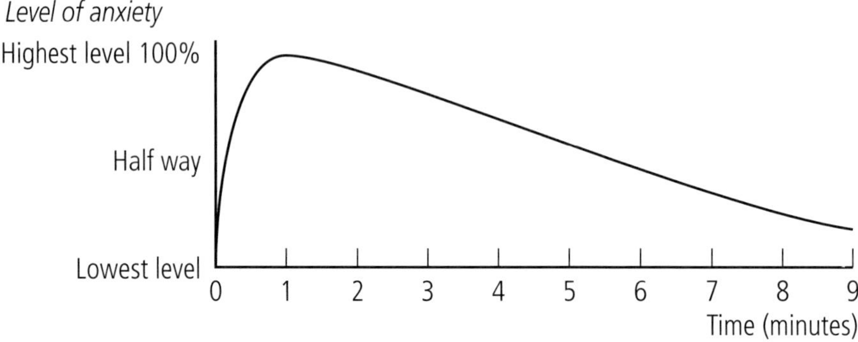

Second time when Paul has a friend round: Wednesday at 11.30am.

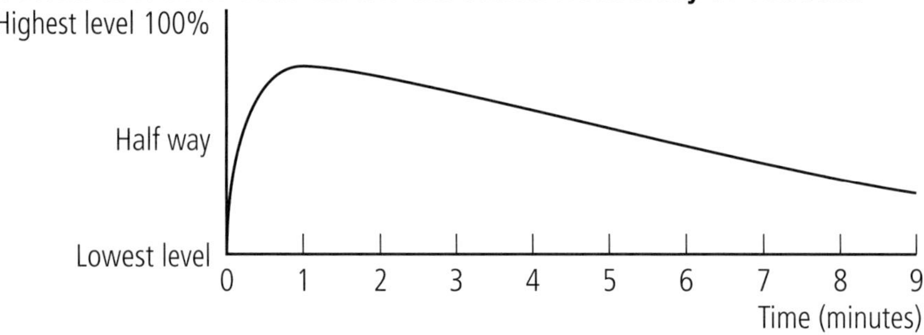

Third time when Paul has a friend round: Friday at 3pm.

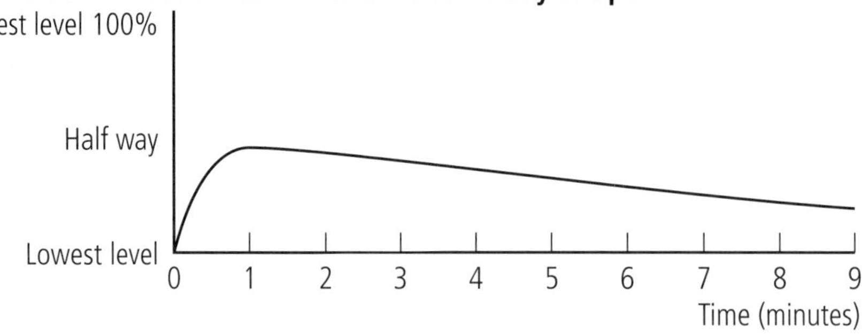

Key point

By facing up to your fears in a planned, step-by-step way, you can overcome them.

Next, think about your **short-term**, **medium-term** and **longer-term** targets.

Example: Paul's short-term, medium-term and longer-term targets

Paul's **short-term plan** over the next week or so: I want to keep meeting up with friends. I also want to push myself by beginning to meet several people together, and do this again and again. In this way I'll start to feel more confident with people.

Paul's **medium-term plan** over the next few weeks: I want to start meeting people I know less well, in groups of two to three people. I also want to go to the photography club in around three weeks' time – perhaps with Raj to start with, so there's a friendly face around. I'll also plan to start talking to people I don't know and saying hello with a big smile on my face and see what happens.

Paul's **longer-term plan** over the next few months: I want to go to the back-to-work course and complete it. I know I'll be anxious to start with – but hopefully I will feel ready for it then. Hopefully it will also lead on to some work afterwards.

Now it's your turn. In creating your plan:

Do:

- Plan to alter **only** one or two things over the next week.
- Plan to slowly alter things in a step-by-step way.
- Use the **questions for effective change** to check that the next step is always well planned.
- Write down your action plan in detail so that you know exactly what to do this week.

Don't:

- Try to alter too many things all at once.
- Choose something that is too hard a target to start with.
- Be negative and think 'It's a waste of time'. Experiment to find out if this negative thinking is actually true.

Your short-term, medium-term and longer-term plans

Your short-term plan – what might you do over the next week or so? This is your next step you need to plan.

Your medium-term plan – what might you aim towards doing over the next few weeks – the next few steps?

Your longer-term plan – where do you want to be in a few months or so?

Remember to plan slow, steady changes. This will help you to rebuild your confidence, as you tackle your avoidance. You'll also probably discover that facing fears is one of the best ways of tackling your worries as well.

Summary

In this workbook you have:

- Found out why we avoid things that seem scary.
- Learned how avoiding things can make you feel worse.
- Made a clear plan to make slow, steady changes to tackle avoidance.
- Planned some next steps to build on this.

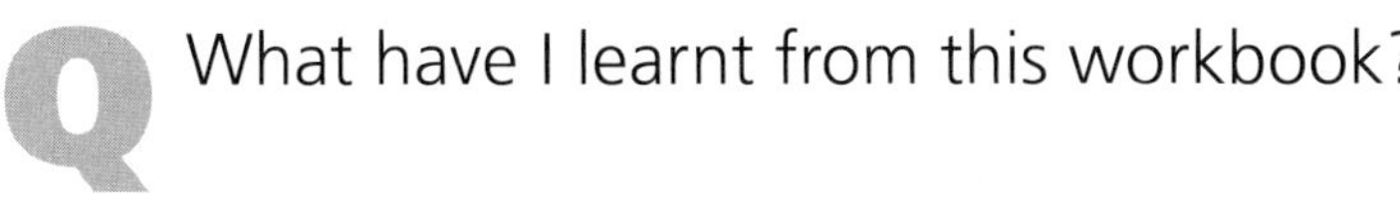

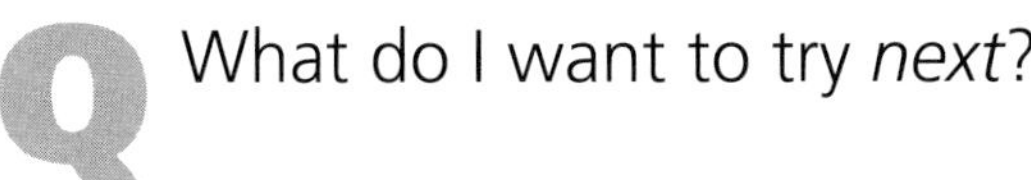

Putting what you have learned into practice

The best way to make changes is by taking slow, steady steps. You're probably a bit fed up with reading this by now but it's true! If at any stage any step seems too much then go back to the drawing board (Step 2) and think up another smaller step you can cope with.

Good luck!

My notes

Overcoming Anxiety, Stress and Panic

A Five Areas Approach

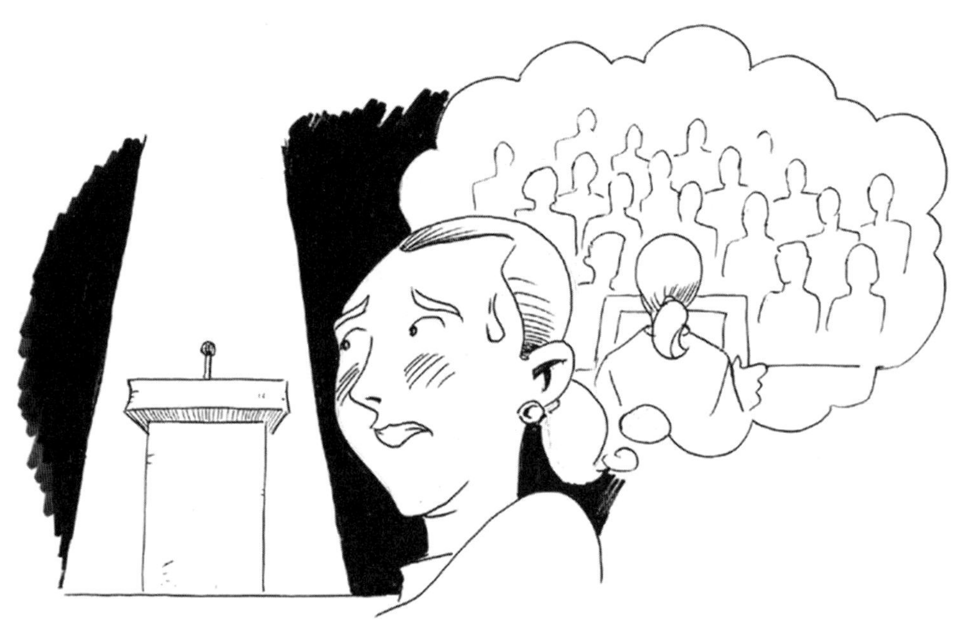

Understanding and overcoming shyness and social phobia

www.livinglifetothefull.com
www.fiveareas.com

Dr Chris Williams

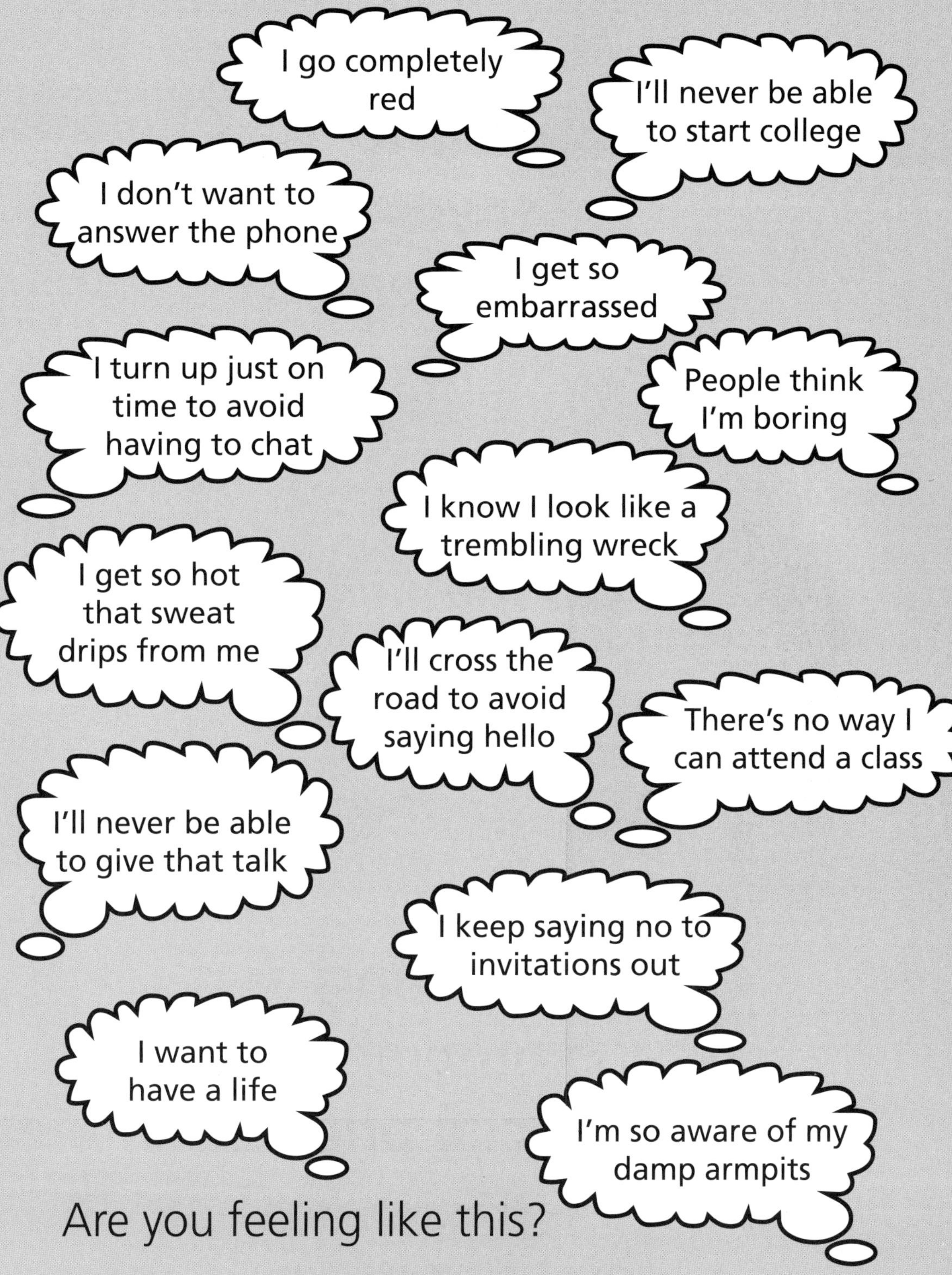
I go completely red
I'll never be able to start college
I don't want to answer the phone
I get so embarrassed
I turn up just on time to avoid having to chat
People think I'm boring
I know I look like a trembling wreck
I get so hot that sweat drips from me
I'll cross the road to avoid saying hello
There's no way I can attend a class
I'll never be able to give that talk
I keep saying no to invitations out
I want to have a life
I'm so aware of my damp armpits

Are you feeling like this?

If so, … this **workbook is for you**.

In this workbook you will:

- Find out how shyness and extreme shyness (social phobia) can affect you.
- Learn how avoiding things can make you feel worse.
- Discover how your anxiety can make you misjudge how you really look and come over to others.
- Make a clear plan to make slow, steady changes to tackle shyness and extreme shyness.
- Plan some next steps to build on this.

How do shyness and extreme shyness (social phobia) affect you?

Many people feel shy to a degree. If you feel shy, you may feel anxious and not at rest or relaxed when meeting new people. Perhaps you have a comfort zone where you feel more relaxed with a few good friends you have known for some time.

Sometimes however, people's anxiety in social situations goes through the roof. *Social phobia* is when a person feels a very high level of anxiety linked to excessive shyness. The person not only feels ill at ease with others – but is also scared of meeting other people. They will go to great lengths to avoid new or uncomfortable social situations. Underlying this is a very strong fear that others are judging them negatively or that they are in some way acting in a deeply humiliating or embarrassing way. This extreme form of shyness affects about one person in 35 at some time in life.

Other situations that people might find difficult include times when others are watching them perform a task, such as giving a talk, dancing or doing karaoke. For example a teacher can become very anxious leading a class. Any other situation where the person is the centre of attention can cause similar symptoms.

Social phobia causes great difficulty in one-to-one situations or whenever the person thinks that the spotlight is on them. For example meeting new people, or making small talk over coffee can seem desperately difficult. Situations such as this lead to *mind-reading* that others don't like you, or judge you to be unattractive, boring, inferior or stupid. These thoughts then further lead to symptoms of strong anxiety. Understandably, this then leads to avoidance of any social situations that cause anxiety.

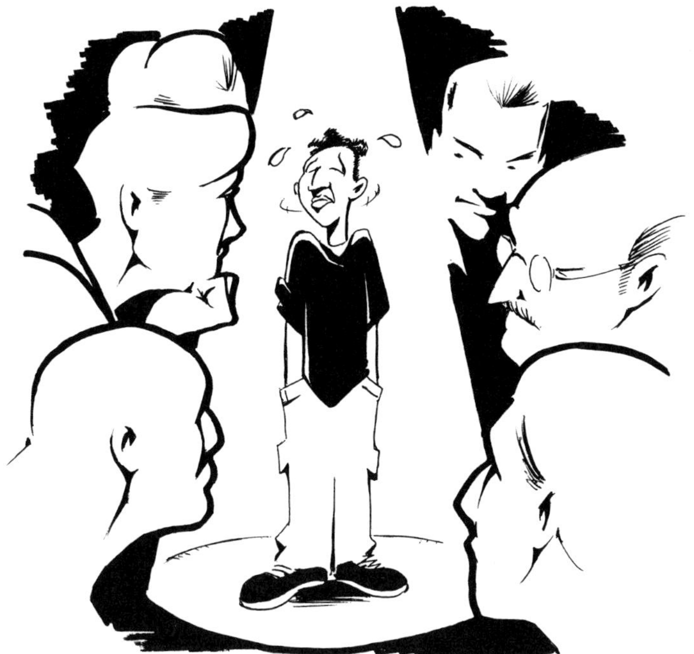

More about phobias

Key point

A *phobia* describes problems of high anxiety (often with panic attacks) that regularly occur in a particular situation. The person becomes overly aware of any possible threats relating to their fear. They try to avoid or quickly leave any situation, people or places that cause them to feel anxious. This happens even though the person often knows logically that the situation will not harm or kill them. Yet they experience the anxiety anyway.

In this chapter to shorten the way problem anxiety and social phobia are described we will talk about *social phobia*.

Let's think about how social anxiety is affecting you.

Social anxiety checklist

Do you notice very strong feelings of anxiety, shame, humiliation, embarrassment or panic when you:

- Talk with one person?

Yes ☐ No ☐ Sometimes ☐

- Join a group of people?

Yes ☐ No ☐ Sometimes ☐

- Give a talk or presentation?

Yes ☐ No ☐ Sometimes ☐

- Dance or perform, for example at a party, or on stage acting?

Yes ☐ No ☐ Sometimes ☐

- Are in situations where there may be physical intimacy/touching/kissing/holding hands/sex?

Yes ☐ No ☐ Sometimes ☐

Q Are you avoiding the above-mentioned situations?

Yes ☐ No ☐ Sometimes ☐

Q Does even thinking about these situations, places or people make you feel nervous?

Yes ☐ No ☐ Sometimes ☐

Q Have you become overly sensitive to anything to do with the activity?

Yes ☐ No ☐ Sometimes ☐

Q Are you downplaying your own ability to overcome these fears?

Yes ☐ No ☐ Sometimes ☐

Q Overall, are you living an increasingly restricted lifestyle as a result?

Yes ☐ No ☐ Sometimes ☐

If you have answered 'Yes' or 'Sometimes' to any of these questions, then it means that social anxiety may be affecting you. Talk to your healthcare practitioner about this to find out if you have social anxiety/shyness or a social phobia.

Key point

Almost everyone is concerned about what people think of them. In many ways that is helpful. If we had no interest in what others thought of us and were only interested in our opinions, we would be potentially very selfish, and certainly very annoying!

Awareness of other people's thoughts about us is needed to allow us all to live together more or less peacefully. Problems arise when these normal social concerns become exaggerated and built up to cause either social anxiety/shyness which distresses you, or a situation where it comes to dominate and ruin your life (social phobia).

Fortunately there are some very good treatments you can use to tackle this anxiety, and reduce the impact on your life.

Now, let's find out more about social anxiety.

Understanding social anxiety using the Five Areas Approach

One helpful way of understanding how social anxiety affects you is to think of the ways that it affects different key areas of your life. The **Five Areas Approach** can help you to do this by looking in detail at five important areas of your life.

The Five Areas are:

- **Area 1: People and events around you**. This area includes the problems you face with talking with **people**, or taking part in certain **events** such as public speaking, dancing or performing. It includes any situations, people or places you find particularly hard to cope with.
- **Area 2: Your thinking**. Your thinking can often become extreme and unhelpful when you feel socially anxious. You worry about how you come over, and are very aware of how you are speaking, acting, dancing or

looking to others. You may mind-read and jump to conclusions that others judge you badly, and that you are performing so poorly it is humiliating. You see yourself as constantly failing against the expectations you set yourself. These scary thoughts cause you to jump to the very worst conclusions. They cause you to feel really bad, and also affect what you do.

- **Area 3: Your feelings (emotions)**. Social anxiety is often mixed with other feelings such as embarrassment or shame. You may feel angry with your own self or others, or feel guilty when you let yourself or others down.
- **Area 4: Altered physical symptoms**. When you feel scared your body also reacts. When you are feeling just a little anxious, you may notice feelings of tension, or you may feel fidgety or find it hard to get off to sleep. When you are feeling even more anxious, you are likely to notice even stronger physical symptoms. You may feel hot, sweaty, shaky or cold, your heart rate goes up and you take rapid shallow breaths, and you may feel dizzy or faint. You may also have an urge to go to the toilet or feel sick. All of these are common symptoms that can happen to anyone at times of anxiety. You can find out more about the wide range of physical symptoms caused by the *fight or flight* adrenaline response in the *Understanding panic and phobias* workbook. For symptoms such as *anxious overbreathing* see the *Overcoming anxious overbreathing (hyperventilation)* workbook.
- **Area 5: Altered behaviour or activity levels**. This includes both – the helpful things you can do to make you feel better, and the unhelpful things you do, which backfire and make you feel even worse.

Now try to think about how the Five Areas assessment can help Dawn understand how she is feeling.

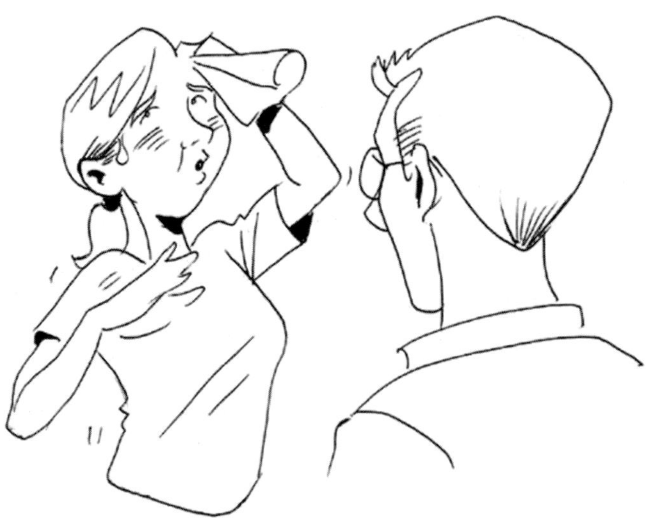

Example: How social anxiety is affecting Dawn's life

Example: Dawn becomes very anxious and scared in social situations. This has worsened since she was a teenager when she had bad acne. Even though the acne has now cleared, her anxiety in social situations has got worse and worse. During these occasions she notices severe physical symptoms of anxiety. She feels hot and flushed, sweaty and slightly shaky. She is very aware of her dry mouth and notices a 'frog' in her throat. Dawn constantly feels that the person she is speaking to will be aware of her discomfort and judge her negatively. She fears looking stupid and small, and mind-reads that others see her as being bright red and very sweaty.

To try to cover these symptoms up she changes what she does by:

- Avoidance: Dawn chooses to avoid social situations where possible. She tends to say no to invitations to meals out or parties, and tries to keep all social encounters as short as possible.
- Unhelpful behaviours: Dawn tries to avoid eye contact with people. She only makes eye contact briefly and for as short a time as possible. She finds herself constantly tempted to cut conversations short and leave abruptly. She is especially aware of feeling hot, flushed and sweaty and uses her handkerchief to repeatedly dab her forehead. She also tries to cool down by fanning herself with her hand and by blowing air from her mouth directed up at her forehead. Finally, she keeps swallowing hard and coughing to try to clear her throat.

So what Dawn **thinks** affects how she **feels** mentally and physically, can also unhelpfully alter what she **does**. Dawn's altered behaviour is designed to help her cope with the anxiety of social contact. But what she doesn't realise is that her actions and avoidance can backfire and undermine her confidence even more.

Hurrying away only strengthens her belief that she can only cope by leaving a situation. Mopping her brow reinforces the fears that others will have judged her negatively. But the actions Dawn takes might actually draw more attention to her as a result. People may ask her if she is feeling okay. This is quite the opposite of what she wished would happen.

The figure below shows how Dawn's problems can be summarised using the Five Areas Approach.

Dawn's Five Areas assessment

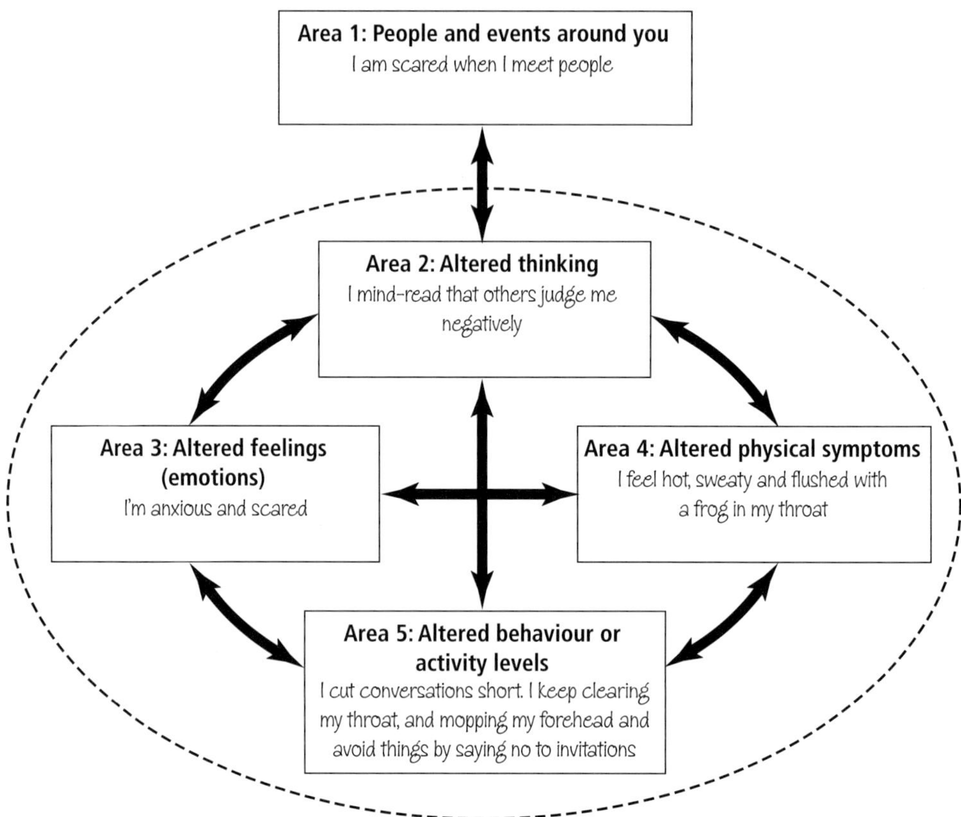

The Five Areas diagram shows that what you think about a situation or problem can affect how you feel physically and mentally. It also shows that your thinking affects what you do (your behaviour or activity levels). Look at the arrows in the diagram. Each of the Five Areas of your life affect each other.

You can find out far more about the Five Areas Approach and how it affects each of the Five Areas in the *Understanding panic and phobias* workbook. For reasons of space this workbook will focus on altered behaviour.

Altered behaviour or activity levels

Some things that you do can worsen how you feel. But many ways in which you respond can be very helpful and boost how you are feeling. The ways in which your altered behaviours may worsen how you feel are:

- Reducing your activity levels by not doing as much as before.
- Avoiding or escaping from doing things that seem scary or too difficult.
- Starting to respond in ways that backfire and make you feel worse.

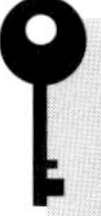

Key point

Making changes in your behaviour and activity levels are some of the most helpful things you can do to boost how you feel.

First type of altered behaviour: Reduced activity

When you feel stressed, tense or down, it's hard to keep doing things because you have:

- Low energy and feel tired ('I'm too tired').
- Little enjoyment or achievement when you do things.
- Negative thoughts about things ('I just can't be bothered').

All these altered behaviours lead to reduced activity – where you do less of or stop doing things **that are important** to you. Often the first things that are squeezed out are those that have previously given you a sense of **fun** or **achievement** (for example, meeting up with friends, and doing things with your family). You can also lose your sense of **closeness** to others.

It begins to feel as though everything is too much effort. And so you feel worse and worse.

Write down any examples of your reduced activities here:

The good news is that once you have noticed whether this is true for you, you can start working on your reduced activity in a planned, step-by-step way. You will find some suggestions for how to do this in the workbook *Facing fears and overcoming avoidance*.

Second type of altered behaviour: Avoiding or escaping from things

People often start to avoid or escape from other people, places and situations that make them feel worried. This may make you feel less anxious in the short term. But in the longer term, avoiding things makes it harder and harder to confidently face your fears in the future. And you don't see that your worst fears don't actually occur. In fact, avoidance teaches people the unhelpful rule that you only coped with a situation by avoiding it.

Key point

Avoidance and escaping can make you feel worse and also undermine your confidence.

Some things you may be avoiding

- Conversations and meeting people.
- Making eye contact – so you look at the floor.
- Joining classes or groups.
- Public performance – for example giving talks, speeches, acting or dancing.
- Generally doing things where you can make mistakes.
- Doing anything that brings attention to you.

Write down any examples of things you have been avoiding here:

Third type of altered behaviour: Dropping helpful things you do

Helpful behaviours include doing things such as:

- Talking to trusted friends or family for support.
- Recognising the times when you have been too hard on yourself.
- Reading or using self-help materials or attending a self-help group.

- Going to see a doctor or healthcare practitioner.
- Finding activities that give you a boost.
- If you have a personal spiritual faith, your beliefs may provide helpful support.

My helpful behaviours

Q Has your social anxiety caused you to stop doing activities that help you?

Yes ☐ No ☐ Sometimes ☐

Write down any examples of helpful behaviours you do here:

> **Key point**
>
> It is important to make time to keep doing these activities as they really do help.

Fourth type of altered behaviour: Unhelpful things you do

Sometimes people may do things that make them feel better at first. But in the longer term, these things backfire and make you feel worse. Do you do any of the following unhelpful behaviours?

1. Trying to escape and hurry away:

- Rushing through difficult situations – for example, talking faster so you can leave quickly.
- Giving only short replies – you try to cut conversations short so you can quickly escape.
- Talking more quickly than normal to get a presentation or talk over with
- Making an excuse, or lying and saying you are ill, or have another urgent reason why you need to leave early or not attend.
- Quickly leaving a place or situation when you feel bad.

2. Distracting yourself mentally by trying hard not to think about how you feel. For example:

- Trying desperately hard not to think about how you feel.
- Trying to block how you feel by doing things that make you feel safer *mentally* (like doing maths sums or saying 'I'm alright' again and again or focusing on the lines on the floor) or through *actions* (such as biting your lip or digging your nails into your hand, gripping hard onto things for support, etc).

These actions backfire on two levels. First, they don't work – and simply stoke up anxiety in the long-term. Second, you will be trying so hard to distract yourself that you won't be focusing on listening, or on performing well. You may come over as distracted and rude, or mess up what you are doing simply because your mind is elsewhere.

3. Blocking how you feel using other approaches:

- Using alcohol or street drugs to block how you feel and to give you false courage.
- Trying very hard to stop shaking – by tensing your muscles. This makes them shake even more.
- Trying to cool yourself, or hide redness, sweat or sweaty armpits. For example by wearing cardigans, fanning or mopping your face, or wafting yourself to cool down. These actions actually backfire by drawing attention to you – because to others you aren't as red, sweaty, etc. as you think you are. Even if you were it doesn't matter – some people just get more hot than others. Interestingly, a well-known teacher and researcher in social phobia encourages people he works with to experiment by pouring water onto their faces, and onto their shirts under their arms so they appear soaking. People are encouraged to wear a blue shirt as this shows up the 'sweat' (water) especially well. They are then encouraged to go and chat to someone and see if any comments are made. The amount of water poured on is far more than anyone would sweat. Usually no one comments. If they do, then the person just says, 'I spilled some water', and no-one is bothered after that. This sort of experiment is very helpful to challenge your worst fears that others will react with shock, criticism or disappointment if you are hot or sweaty.
- Misusing prescribed medication by taking extra doses that are not prescribed to block how you feel.

Other unhelpful behaviours are:

- Withdrawing into yourself and cutting yourself off from your friends or family.
- Neglecting yourself (for example, by not eating as much or not washing).
- Finding yourself tempted to do things that you know are unwise or wrong. This might include deliberately taking risks or picking fights.
- Harming yourself as a way of blocking how you feel (for example, self-cutting).
- Shouting or screaming at others out of frustration or getting angry if people seem to crowd you.

Write down any examples of unhelpful behaviour you do here:

The purpose of all the unhelpful behaviours is to feel safer/better – at least in the short term. Therefore they are sometimes called *safety* behaviours. But, although safety behaviours may help you feel better in the short term, this doesn't last. **The anxiety returns to the same or even higher level**. For example, drinking too much alcohol or taking sedative drugs may give you a sense of false courage, but such things lead to more problems of their own.

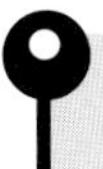

Key point

An important thing to watch out for is whether you have got into a habit of reacting to difficult situations in certain ways. By watching out for any unhelpful behaviours that you may have a tendency to fall into, and by choosing to respond differently, you can make large changes to how you are feeling.

What next?

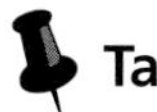

Task

Now test out how accurate your fears are by seeing how others and you react when you, for example, talk, make eye contact or dance. The *Noticing and changing anxious thinking* workbook will help you tackle these fears. In particular, it is worth being aware of some of the main things that happen:

- You jump to the worst conclusions and catastrophise that you are performing terribly. You feel this way, even though others don't see it that way. For example, you are likely to see yourself as being redder, more sweaty, flustered, bumbling, unable to talk, clumsy and odd looking than real life. These fears are built up by your own inner fears. They are reinforced by how you feel physically. Anxiety causes you to feel hot, flushed and sweaty. You can test out whether others are that bothered by this by facing your fears.
- You feel fearful of making mistakes. By choosing to introduce small errors into what you do, you can again test out exactly what happens if things aren't done perfectly. Usually things done 'good enough' are literally that good enough.

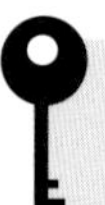

Key point

The best way to tackle your anxious fears is to act against them in a planned, step-by-step way.

Seven steps to tackling avoidance

You may have tried to stop avoiding things before. But unless you have a clear plan and stick to it, change will be hard to make. Making one change at a time is the main thing that will help you move forwards. This may mean choosing at first **not** to focus on other areas.

By setting targets you can focus on how to make the changes needed to get better. To do this, you need to decide your:

- **Short-term targets** – these are the changes you can make today, tomorrow and in the next week.
- **Medium-term targets** – these are the changes to be put in place over the next few weeks.
- **Long-term targets** – this is where you want to be in six months or a year's time.

By working through the seven steps below you can learn how to plan clear ways of overcoming avoidance. The aim is to slowly plan **specific** activities to boost your confidence and tackle avoidance. The good news is that you plan this one step at a time. And you can keep practising a step until you feel comfortable at that step. That way it never seems too much or too scary.

Step 1: Identify and clearly define your problem

The following checklist gives the activities that are commonly avoided when people are anxious socially. You will probably have noticed avoiding at least some of these activities.

Checklist: Identifying your patterns of worsening avoidance

As a result of how you feel are you:	Tick here if you have noticed this – even if just sometimes
Avoiding talking to others face to face?	☐
Avoiding being in situations where you may need to talk/do things with others?	☐
Not making eye contact – so you look at the floor?	☐
Not joining classes or groups?	☐
Not participating in public performance – for example giving talks, speeches, acting or dancing?	☐
Generally, doing things where you can make mistakes?	☐
Doing things that don't bring attention to you?	☐
Putting off dealing with important practical problems (both large and small)?	☐
Not really being honest with others?	
For example, saying 'Yes' when you really mean 'No' or by not saying things that you really want to	☐
Avoiding answering the phone, or the door when people visit?	☐
Avoiding physical intimacy or having sex because of anxiety?	☐

Write down any other activities you are avoiding here:

Example: Paul's avoidance

Paul has been invited to join a back-to-work course that starts in four weeks. He feels very anxious about going and fears he will go red and start stuttering. But he knows he needs to go to the course to help him rebuild his confidence.

Choosing a first target

Now it's your turn. Use the list above to choose a single target that you will focus on to start with. This is particularly important if you have ticked several boxes in the checklist. It isn't possible to work on all these areas at once. Instead you need to decide which **one** area to focus on to start with.

Example: Paul breaks his target into smaller steps

Paul wants to attend the back-to-work course. This starts in four weeks' time. Paul decides he needs to start building his confidence up towards getting there. He has realised that he tries to avoid talking to people, even to the extent of crossing the road if he sees someone ahead he knows.

Paul therefore decides to focus on something that would be a good first step towards getting to the course – building confidence when he's talking to others. This is something that would help tackle a big problem for him – which is affecting whether he can go on the course.

Paul's target: *I'm going to focus on feeling more comfortable talking to others.*

Write down one problem you want to work on here. (Remember that this should be a thing you are avoiding.)

Be a detective

The next thing is to do some research on your avoidance. First, record in detail every time you avoid your chosen problem over several days. At the back of the workbook in the My notes section write down:

- What you avoid.
- When you avoid it.
- How much you do it (for example, don't go out, don't go to the shops, don't say hello – because of worries).
- How long it lasts for.

Well done! Now try to understand more about your avoidance and why you tend to do it. Try to work out why you avoid or escape from things such as:

- The time of day.
- Whether you slept well the night before.
- Who you were with and how they responded.
- What went through your mind.
- How you felt emotionally and physically at the time.
- Any other things you did to try to cope or escape.

... and anything else that seems to help explain your reaction.

Write any important things you have learned here:

Check point: is your target a realistic target? Answer the **Questions for change** to find out:

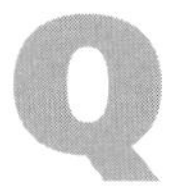

Is your target:

- Clear and realistic and something that you can tackle over the next week or two?

  Yes ☐ No ☐

- Not so scary that you can't face doing it?

  Yes ☐ No ☐

- Still helping you move forwards?

  Yes ☐ No ☐

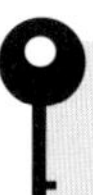

Key point

Sometimes you need to make sure that your first target really is a small, focused problem so that you can tackle it in one step.

Now use your notes to decide if you need to break down your avoidance behaviour into smaller steps that you can target one at a time.

Q Do you need to break the avoidance down into a number of smaller, more achievable targets?

Yes ☐ No ☐

If you answered 'No', then please go straight to Step 2. If you answered 'Yes', then make sure you've chosen a new, smaller and realistic first target and write it here.

My clear first step is:

Step 2: Think up as many solutions as possible to achieve your initial target

Try to come up with as many ideas as possible. Include completely whacky ideas in your list as well, even if you wouldn't choose to do them. This will help you to **think broadly**. Here are some useful questions to help you to think up possible solutions:

- What advice would you give a friend who was trying to tackle the same problem?
- What ridiculous solutions can you include as well as more sensible ones?
- What helpful suggestions would others make?
- How could you look at the solutions facing you differently? What would you have said before you felt like this, or what might you say about the situation, say in five years' time?
- What approaches have you tried in the past in similar circumstances?

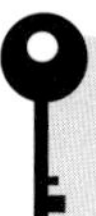

Key point

If you feel stuck, sometimes doing this task with someone you trust can help.

Example: Paul's ideas

I could:

- Pay an actor to be my friend and talk to me. I'd feel in charge then!
- Start small – and build up my confidence on the phone.
- Ask a friend to come round to chat so that I can practise talking again with someone who I know likes me.
- Start going again to the photography club I used to attend.

Now write down as many possible options (including ridiculous ideas at first) for your own situation:

Step 3: Look at the pros and cons of each possible solution

Example: Paul's list of pros and cons

Idea	Pros (advantages)	Cons (disadvantages)
Pay an actor to be my friend and talk to me. I'd feel in charge then!	They'd be there all day. I could ask them to be friendly and nice	That's a crazy idea. But wouldn't it be great to have that much money!
Start small – and build up my confidence on the phone	This is a small step which is great	I'm actually okay on the phone. It's more when I actually am with someone that I start to go red and clam up
Ask a friend to come round to chat so that I can practise talking again with someone who I know likes me	That sounds perfect. If it's someone I trust it wouldn't matter to me as much as someone who's not a friend. I could do that and I think it would help me build my confidence again	I might clam up. But then I don't think that should happen. I just need to plan a few conversation starters for if things go quiet. I think that's okay
Start going again to the photography club I used to attend	Wouldn't that be great! I could go in and suddenly be confident all over again with people I know	It just doesn't seem that realistic. It's too big a step. I'd turn up and just sit alone in the corner embarrassed. Or I'd leave and never go back

Write your own list of ideas into the following table, along with the pros and cons of each suggestion.

My suggestions from Step 2	Pros (advantages)	Cons (disadvantages)

Step 4: Now choose one of the solutions

Choose a solution that is a small step in the right direction and you think will be likely to succeed. Look at the list you made in Step 3 to help you with this.

The best way to tackle avoidance is to plan **steady, slow changes**. In this way, you can rebuild your confidence. The step should be small enough to be possible, but big enough to move you forwards.

Example: Paul's choice

Paul decides to ask his friend Raj to come round to chat so that he can practise talking again with someone he knows he gets on with.

Write your choice here:

Now check your choice against some of the **Questions for effective change**.

Q Will your chosen step be useful for changing how you are?

Yes ☐ No ☐

Q Is it a specific task so that you will know when you've done it?

Yes ☐ No ☐

Q Is it realistic, practical and achievable?

Yes ☐ No ☐

If you answered 'Yes' to all three questions your chosen step should help start you off. If you can't answer 'Yes' to all three questions at the moment, rewrite your plan until you can.

Step 5: Plan the steps needed to carry it out

You need to have a clear plan that will help you to decide exactly **what** you are going to do and **when** you are going to do it. **Write down** the steps needed to carry out your plan. This will help you to think what to do and also think of the possible problems that might arise. An important part of the plan is to try to think what could block the plan from happening or make it hard for you to follow it. That way you can think about how you would respond to keep your plan on track.

Example: Paul's plan

Paul phones his friend Raj, whom he knows from way back at school. They have stayed in close touch since and remain good friends. Raj knows Paul has struggled with depression. But Paul hasn't seen Raj for a few weeks and is a little nervous about how things will go. He therefore decides the following plan: 'Raj will come by at 3 o'clock tomorrow. We can have a cup of tea or coffee and have a chat. If it's good weather we could walk and talk.'

Paul also tries to think of what might go wrong or cause problems. He thinks he may feel uncomfortable about silences. Therefore he plans to make sure he has a few questions to use to get things going if needed. He looks through the hints and tips for starting and keeping conversations going in the *How to ask for what you really need (being assertive)* workbook. Now he feels confident Raj and he will have enough things to talk about.

Now write down your plan here:

What if you think that there's something that may block your plan? Write down what you could do next to unblock it.

Now check your plan against the rest of the **Questions for effective change**:

Q Does your plan make clear what you are going to do and when you are going to do it?

Yes ☐ No ☐

Q Is it an activity that won't be easily blocked or prevented by practical problems?

Yes ☐ No ☐

Q Will it help you to learn useful things even if it doesn't work out perfectly?

Yes ☐ No ☐

Step 6: Carry out the plan

Your task now is to carry out your plan during the next week.

As you get ready to put your plan into action be aware of worrying thoughts or fears. One of the best ways of checking how true unhelpful fears are is to act against them and see what happens.

Pay attention to any thoughts and fears you may have about what will happen before, during and after you have completed your plan. Write any thoughts/fears you noticed here:

If things seem just too scary, plan that you will carry out the plan *anyway* and see what happens. If things do seem too scary, then go back to Step 2 (your brainstorm) and pick something that is a less scary first step.

Good luck!

Step 7: Review the outcome

Example: Paul's review

Raj is a little late, which makes Paul feel slightly more nervous. He starts making the tea to keep busy. When Raj arrives, Paul is no longer that anxious and they start chatting straight away.

Later, Paul thinks that Raj's visit helped a lot. He also thinks that when he finally gets to the course, he should remember that doing something while waiting helps. Paul really enjoyed the chat with Raj.

Well done on carrying out your plan. Now write down your own review here:

Q Was your plan successful?

Yes ☐ No ☐

Q Did it help improve things?

Yes ☐ No ☐

Q Did any problems arise?

Yes ☐ No ☐

Things that can de-rail your plans

When you feel anxious, there are three common behaviours that can act to keep you feeling anxious and stop you improving.

As a result of how you feel, do you:	Tick here if you have noticed this – even if just sometimes
1. Hurry through your plan and try to leave/escape quickly For example: walking or talking faster, cutting things short, making your excuses and leaving, or even lying that you need to be elsewhere or feel ill	☐
2. Do things that make you feel safer in the short term For example: misusing medication, drink or street drugs to give you false courage and block how you feel	☐
3. Try hard to distract yourself from fearful or worrying thoughts or physical symptoms For example: trying to say positive comments again and again ('I'll be alright, I'll be alright'); trying hard to think of something else (such as counting the tiles on a wall); doing something physical to hurt or distract you from fears (such as clenching your fists, biting your lip, digging your nails into your hand)	☐

Each of the above three behaviours seems very attractive at the time. However, they are all ways of *subtle avoidance*. They make you feel better – at the time. But in the long-term they can actually worsen how you feel.

If you have noticed that your plan hasn't gone as well as you hoped, check if any of these three behaviours have de-railed you. If so, you need to take what happened into account when you plan the next step.

What have you learned from doing this?

Write down any helpful lessons or information you have learned from what happened. If things didn't go quite as you hoped, try to learn from what happened.

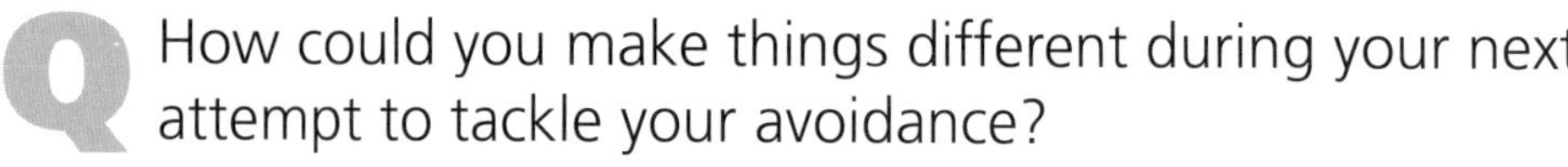

How could you make things different during your next attempt to tackle your avoidance?

Were you too ambitious in choosing the target you did?

Planning the next steps

Now that you have reviewed how your first planned target went, the next step is to plan another change to build on this. You will need to slowly build on what you have done in a step-by-step way.

You have the choice to:

- Stick with the target you have achieved.
- Focus on the same problem area and plan to keep working on this.
- Choose a new area to work on.

There are pros and cons of each of these choices. Think about these when you make your choice.

When you are making this decision, bear in mind that by practising the same step **again and again** over the next few weeks your confidence will grow. Your anxious fears will also get less and last for a shorter and shorter time.

This happens no matter what fear you try to tackle. Facing up to a fear causes it to slowly lose its effect on you. Look at how Paul's fear has reduced.

First time Paul has a friend round: Tuesday at 3pm.

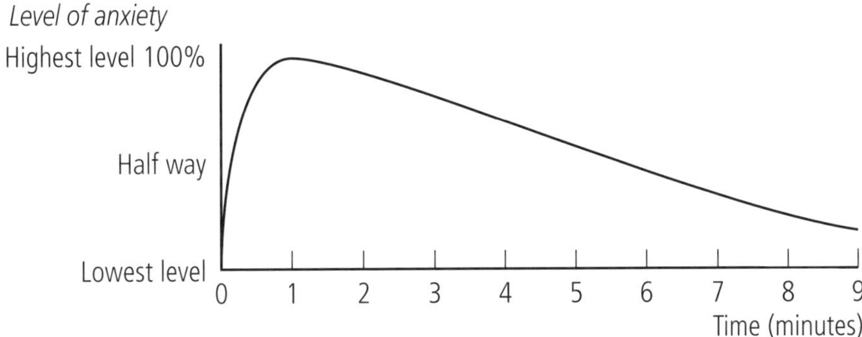

Second time when Paul has a friend round: Wednesday at 11.30am.

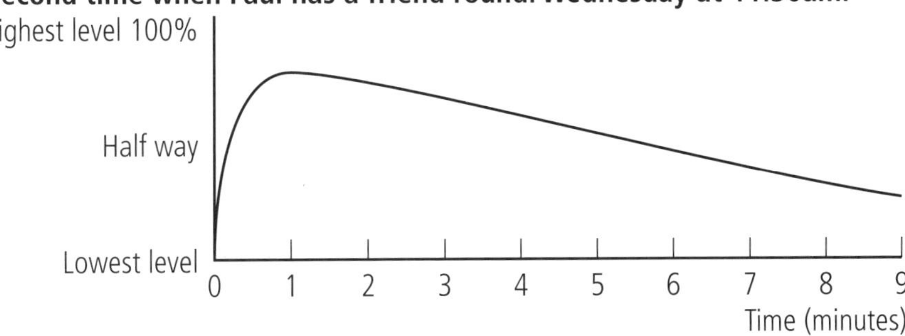

Third time when Paul has a friend round: Friday at 3pm.

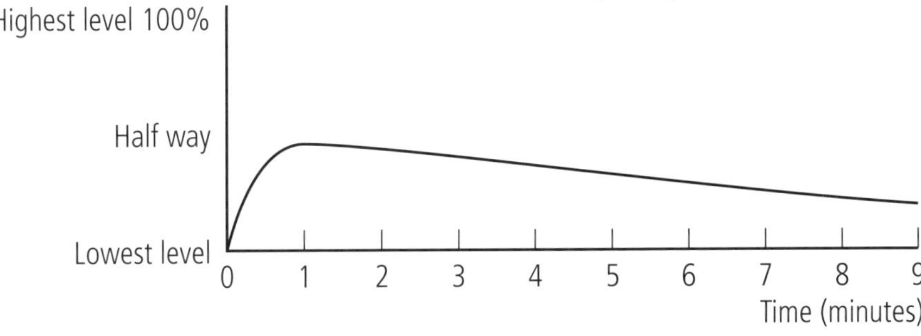

Key point

By facing up to your fears in a planned, step-by-step way, you can overcome them.

Next, think about your **short-term**, **medium-term** and **longer-term** targets.

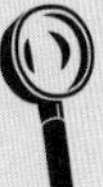

Example: Paul's short-term, medium-term and longer-term targets

Paul's **short-term plan** over the next week or so: *I want to keep meeting up with friends. I also want to push myself by beginning to meet several people together, and do this again and again. In this way I'll start to feel more confident with people.*

Paul's **medium-term plan** over the next few weeks: *I want to start meeting people I know less well, in groups of two to three people. I also want to go to the photography club in around three weeks' time. I'll also plan to start talking to people I don't know and saying hello with a big smile on my face and see what happens.*

Paul's **longer-term plan** over the next few months: *I want to go to the back-to-work course and complete it. I know I'll be anxious to start with – but hopefully I will feel ready for it then. Hopefully it will also lead on to some work afterwards.*

Now it's your turn. In creating your plan:

Do:

- Plan to alter **only** one or two things over the next week.
- Plan to slowly alter things in a step-by-step way.
- Use the **questions for effective change** to check that the next step is always well planned.
- Write down your action plan in detail so that you know exactly what to do this week.

Don't:

- Try to alter too many things all at once.
- Choose something that is too hard a target to start with.
- Be negative and think 'It's a waste of time'. Experiment to find out if this negative thinking is actually true.

Your short-term, medium-term and longer-term plans

Your short-term plan – what might you do over the next week or so? This is your next step you need to plan.

Your medium-term plan – what might you aim towards doing over the next few weeks – the next few steps?

Your longer-term plan – where do you want to be in a few months or so?

Remember to plan slow, steady changes. This will help you to rebuild your confidence, as you tackle your avoidance. You'll also probably discover that facing fears is one of the best ways of tackling your worries as well.

Additional useful things to consider

Some tasks that can be useful when planning to overcome problems of social phobia are given here.

- **Learn useful techniques for small talk**. There are several ways to keep the other person talking. Plan a series of questions you can ask when the conversation seems to flag. These can include questions starting Why, What, Where, When, How. For example, *How* was your holiday? *Why* did you choose to go to Turkey? *Where* did you stay? *What* was the beach like? etc. The same five questions can help you to small talk your way around any topic. Remember to allow the person to answer. Don't interrupt them or cut them off. Also listen to what they say. Don't spend so much time rehearsing your next question that you overlook that they have already answered it.
- **Learn how to look just past people**. If you find that making eye contact with people is difficult, then practise looking into the middle distance just past their heads. For example look at a picture on a wall just behind the person, but in a way that it appears that you are looking at them. Practise making brief eye contact and gradually increase the amount and length of this.
- **Role-play**. A good way of reducing anxiety in social situations is to practise small talk with someone you trust. For example, ask a friend to help you to practise conversations. A number of self-help groups also offer regular drop-in classes or specific classes for people with social phobia. Consider attending an anxiety management group. Everyone else there will also have problems with anxiety, and this could be built in as part of your own plan of self-treatment.
- **Video yourself talking to others**. This will provide you with powerful feedback and allow you to test out fears that you are dripping with sweat, shaking like a leaf, or look in some way 'odd'. It will also help you to check out how others react to you. You could do this yourself with a friend if you have access to a video. Healthcare practitioners sometimes offer this approach if you jointly agree that it will be helpful.

Be sure to try to reduce or act against subtle avoidance as part of your plan. For example:

- Relax your posture and allow yourself to move/walk more freely.
- Relax your hands rather than gripping them tightly etc.
- Finally, **watch your alcohol intake**. Make sure you don't use alcohol as a means of building false confidence with other people. This will just add to your problems.

Sources of extra help

You can ask:

- **Your family doctor or GP**. Your GP can offer medical advice and (if they feel it is necessary) refer you to a mental health specialist for a detailed assessment.

Other organisations you can approach are:

- Anxiety UK: this charity has excellent online resources at **www.anxietyuk.org.uk**. There are forums and live chat as well as email support. The charity also has a helpline (**08444 775 774** – Monday to Friday 9.30 am–5.30 pm).
- Triumph over Phobia: this charity runs local groups for people with anxiety, panic and obsessive-compulsive problems. (See **www.topuk.org** or call 0845 600 9601 or email: **info@topuk.org**)

Summary

In this workbook you have:

- Discovered how shyness and extreme shyness (social phobia) affect you.
- Learned how avoiding things can make you feel worse.
- Discovered how your anxiety makes you misjudge how you really look and come across to others.
- Made a clear plan to make slow, steady changes to tackle extreme shyness.
- Planned some next steps to build on this.

What have I learnt from this workbook?

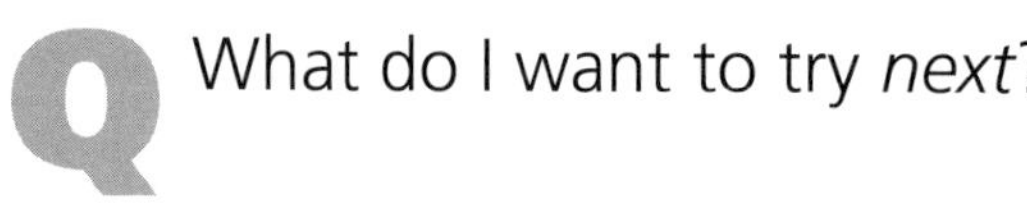

Putting what you have learned into practice

The best way to make changes is by taking slow, steady steps. You're probably a bit fed up with reading this by now but it's true! If at any stage any step seems too much then go back to the drawing board (Step 2) and think up another smaller step you can cope with.

Good luck!

My notes

Overcoming Anxiety, Stress and Panic
A Five Areas Approach

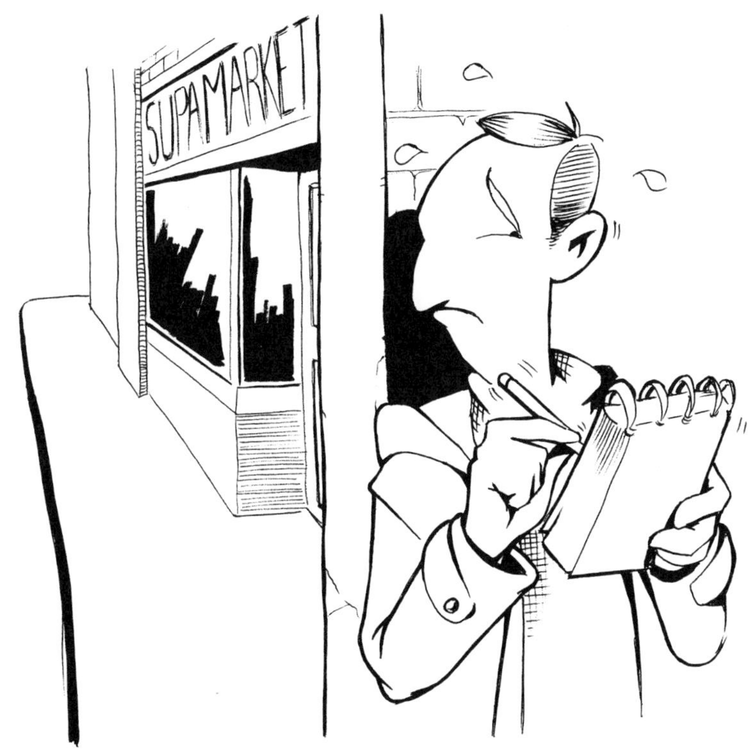

Noticing and changing anxious thinking

www.livinglifetothefull.com
www.fiveareas.com

Dr Chris Williams

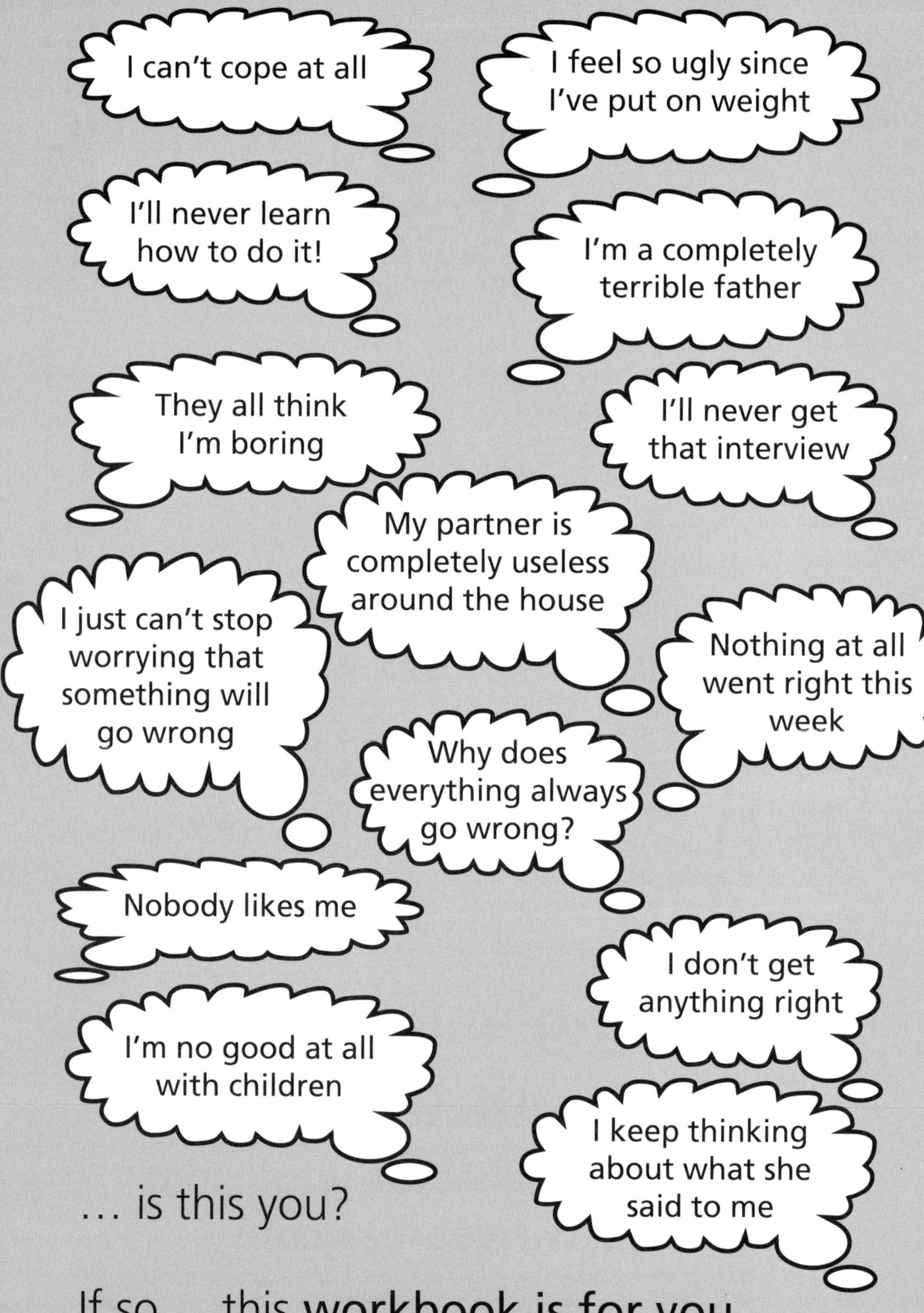
I can't cope at all
I feel so ugly since I've put on weight
I'll never learn how to do it!
I'm a completely terrible father
They all think I'm boring
I'll never get that interview
My partner is completely useless around the house
I just can't stop worrying that something will go wrong
Nothing at all went right this week
Why does everything always go wrong?
Nobody likes me
I don't get anything right
I'm no good at all with children
I keep thinking about what she said to me
... is this you?

If so ... this **workbook is for you**.

When you feel anxious, panicky or low you can:

- Have worrying and fearful thoughts – these make you **tense and stressed**.
- Have unhappy, negative thoughts – these can make you feel **low and sad**.
- Have frustrated, angry thoughts about yourself, your situation and sometimes about others such as your partner, children, friends and relatives. These can make you more **irritable or ratty**.

You could have **all sorts of upsetting thoughts** about how you feel, your current situation and your future outlook.

In this workbook you will learn:

- How to recognise patterns of anxious thinking that worsen how you feel.
- How to respond to upsetting thoughts in ways that help.
- How to change this sort of thinking so it's less upsetting.

The first step in changing anxious thinking is to start noticing how **common** it is in your life.

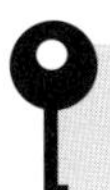

Key point

Anxiety, worry, stress, panic, frustration, anger, irritability, distress, shame, guilt and feeling down are often linked to unhelpful thinking.

Going through the checklist below will help you to recognise whether your thinking is unhelpful.

Checklist: The unhelpful thinking styles

Unhelpful thinking style	Some typical thoughts	Tick if you have noticed this thinking style recently – even if it's just sometimes
Being your own worst critic/bias against yourself	• I'm very self-critical • I overlook my strengths • I see myself as not coping • I don't recognise my achievements • I knew that would happen to me!	☐ ☐ ☐ ☐ ☐
Putting a negative slant on things (negative mental filter)	• I see things through dark, tinted glasses • I see the glass as being half empty rather than half full • Whatever I've done it's never enough to give me a sense of achievement • I tend to focus on the bad side of everyday situations	☐ ☐ ☐ ☐
Having a gloomy view of the future (making negative predictions)	• Things will stay bad or just get worse • Things will go wrong • I'm always expecting to fail	☐ ☐ ☐
Jumping to the very worst conclusion (catastrophising)	• I tend to think that the very worst outcome will happen • I often think that I will fail badly	☐ ☐
Having a negative view about how others see me (mind-reading)	• I often think that others don't like me or think badly of me without any reason for it	☐
Unfairly taking responsibility for things	• I feel guilty about things even if they aren't really my fault. I think I'm responsible for everyone else	☐

➜

Unhelpful thinking style	Some typical thoughts	Tick if you have noticed this thinking style recently – even if it's just sometimes
Making extreme statements or rules	• I use the words 'always' and 'never' a lot	☐
	• If one bad thing happens to me I often say 'just typical' because it seems this *always* happens	☐
	• I make myself a lot of 'must', 'should', 'ought' or 'got to' rules	☐

Almost everyone has these sorts of thoughts each and every day. This doesn't mean that:

- You think like this **all** the time.
- You have to notice **all** of the unhelpful thinking styles.

However, unhelpful thinking can affect how you feel.

Where do unhelpful thoughts come from?

While growing up, people learn how to relate to others from their parents, teachers and friends. Most of us are also influenced by other things such as TV and magazines. But these often portray a picture of perfection that is impossible to live up to in the real world.

Many people mentally beat themselves up over things they *must/should/ought* to do, or over things they think they haven't done well. So you often overlook that you are doing a far better job than you are giving yourself credit for. It can be very hard to live up to these sorts of standards – which can make you stressed and upset. You can also learn to respond in other quite unhelpful ways, which worsens how you feel and affects what you do. **Most often the unhelpful thinking styles are wrong as well as unhelpful.**

Example: Common worries and fears

- **Worrying about what people think of you**
  A common worry that people have is that other people think negatively about them (e.g. that they find you boring or don't want to talk to you). This can make you feel nervous with others, avoid conversations or become distracted or worried as you talk. By acting *against* this fear you can begin to discover that most people have no such thoughts and are happy to chat with you.

- **Fear of fainting or collapsing**
  A very common fear during panic is that you are going to collapse or faint. In fact, people faint or pass out when their heart rate slows, and they don't have enough blood coming to their head. Everything goes quite distant and they fall to the floor. This is a protective action by your body to allow blood to get to your head.

  But exactly the opposite happens during panic. More than enough blood is pumped to the brain (your heart is beating quickly). Rather than things going distant, you are more than painfully aware of how bad you feel. It is the anxious over-breathing (see below) that causes the feelings of dizziness that convince you that you will fall over. The key is to slow down your breathing, close your mouth and take normal-sized slower breaths.

- **Fear of having a heart attack**
  When people get scared, their heart beats faster. You can also become aware of pain in the chest (either because of over-breathing or because of increased tightness in the muscles between the ribs). You then become overly focused on the pain and the anxiety speeds up your heart. This in turn convinces you that you are dying of a heart attack – and worsens the entire scary cycle. As for fear of fainting, again, the real cause is panic and anxiety.

- **Fear of suffocating**
  Another common fear that occurs during times of anxious over-breathing is that you will suffocate. Because both your heart rate and breathing rate increase rapidly, your body and brain are getting more than enough oxygen. But a chemical reaction occurs because of the fast shallow breaths. A gas called carbon dioxide is breathed away, causing you to feel

➜

dizzy with tingling in your body. You also feel a strange sensation of being short of breath. You can find out more about how to deal with this in the *Overcoming anxious overbreathing (hyperventilation)* workbook.

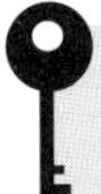

Key point

Often these sorts of scary physical symptoms worsen your fears – when in fact the symptoms are simply unpleasant but not dangerous.

How does unhelpful thinking affect you?

Often people believe in unhelpful kinds of thoughts just because they 'feel' true. This is a result of how you're feeling in yourself. And you can often forget to check out how true these thoughts really are.

Usually these kinds of thoughts can make you feel a little upset, but then you quickly move on and get on with life. But there are times when you're more prone to these thoughts and find them harder to dismiss. For example, when you have some problem you're finding hard to cope with, or if you're distressed and worn down. At times like this, you may also dwell on such thoughts more than usual. And you may find it harder to move on.

Remember that what you think can have a powerful effect on how you **feel** and what you **do**. So unhelpful thinking can lead to:

1. **Mood changes** – you may become more anxious, down, guilty, upset, anxious, ashamed, panicky, stressed or angry.
2. **Behaviour changes** – you may stop doing things or avoid doing things that seem scary. Or you may end up reacting in ways that backfire, such as pushing others away or even drinking too much or using street drugs to cope.

The result is that unhelpful thinking styles worsen how you feel.

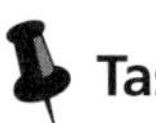

Task

The following table shows the links between your thoughts, feelings and behaviour. You'll notice in the last column of the table there is a suggestion that stopping, thinking and reflecting (**before** getting carried away by the thought and just ending up feeling worse) could help you feel better.

Example: The effect of your thinking on how you feel and what you do

People and events around us	Unhelpful thinking style	Altered feelings and physical sensations	Altered behaviour
You are walking down the road and someone you know walks past and says nothing. She doesn't smile or meet your eye – just walks by Thought: *Irina doesn't like me*	This is an unhelpful thinking style: mind-reading (that Irina doesn't like you); jumping to the worst conclusion; being your own worst critic; being biased against your own self	Low/down and upset; anxious in case you meet again	Feel so down you just go home; avoid Irina in future. **Stop, think and reflect**: *You never checked out that this was the real reason. Maybe Irina just didn't see you?*
You are walking down the road and someone you know walks past and says nothing. She doesn't smile or meet your eye – just walks by Thought: *There's poor Irina – she looks really distracted and upset. I hope she's okay*	This is normal concern for others. It isn't an unhelpful thinking style	Concern for Irina	You turn round and catch up with Irina to say hello. Irina looks a little surprised to begin with and says she didn't see you. You get chatting and have a really nice talk. Irina has been going through a tough time recently. At the end you both agree to meet for lunch after shopping to catch up. **Stop, think and reflect**: *I'm really pleased I spoke to her. She is feeling upset. It was nice to talk – and she seemed pleased too. She suggested we meet up for lunch, which is good because it says to me that she wants to see me and enjoyed chatting*

People and events around us	Unhelpful thinking style	Altered feelings and physical sensations	Altered behaviour
You are at a supermarket checkout trying to pack your bags. You hear someone behind you tut. Thought: *I'm being too slow. They're annoyed with me*	This is another unhelpful thinking style: being your own worst critic; as well as mind-reading that people are irritated by your slowness	Anxiety; perhaps irritated – how dare they – I'm trying my hardest!	**If anxious**: maybe speed up packing – fumble and start to drop things. Make all sorts of apologies **If irritated**: perhaps slow down the packing,stare at them or pass a sarcastic comment which backfires because you end up in an argument **Stop, think and reflect**: *Maybe they were tutting at something else. Maybe they'd forgotten to pick up the apples. Maybe their teeth don't fit!*
You are walking in the countryside on a popular walk when you get to a footbridge over a fast-moving river. The bridge seems well built but has some three-centimetre gaps between the planks on the walkway, and you can see the river below Thought: *I can't walk on that. What If I slip through and fall – or one of the planks is rotten and breaks?* You have asked yourself some questions here: '*What if I slip through and fall or one of the planks is rotten and breaks*'? In answering this question another fear pops into your mind: *'I'll fall and be swept away; I'll drown'*	These thoughts are scary (catastrophic), and also show a bias against yourself (that you can't walk over a safe-looking bridge) Your fears also vastly over estimate how likely it is you will fall and die from a bridge which is on a popular walk and will be well maintained	Anxiety and fear at a very high level. Rapid heart rate and breathing – feel terrified. This sort of intense fear of heights is called a *phobia* In psychiatry books phobias are often described as being excessive and irrational fears. In fact mostly these are learned fears. The fears often link to other concerns	You may refuse to cross the bridge and go back the way you came. Or choose a completely different route and end up going miles out of your way. This may be embarrassing for you and irritating for others you are with **Stop, think and reflect**: *Is it really likely that this bridge – that looks well-maintained – would break? It's a popular walk, and there's no sign the planks are damaged. I'm overestimating how likely this is to happen. The only way I can check that out is to cross it. And I'm going to do this at a normal pace – and not run'. This illustrates an important point: sometimes the only way of testing out an extreme fear is to step out and act against it.*

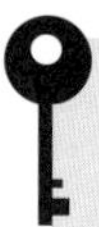

Key point

Thinking in these extreme and anxious ways means that you're only looking at part of the picture. Because of this, these thinking styles are often not true. Remember as in the bridge example in the table: sometimes the only way of testing out an extreme fear is to step out and act against it.

But what if my unhelpful thoughts are true?

Of course some of these thoughts can be true at times. For example, if you have a child, you are responsible for his or her safety and health. But others around you also have a part to play in this. So although you are responsible most of the time, it becomes unhelpful if you focus on your negative thoughts and feel crushed by them.

The same is true for the other types of thoughts. Sometimes when you mind-read, you are right – someone you know may not like you. Sometimes you may annoy another person by your packing, or a bridge may really be dangerous. But remember that when you feel stressed or low you worry too much about these things, and jump to conclusions about how badly wrong they may go.

Being aware that most people are prone to thinking in this way at some time – and even more so when feeling stressed, anxious, low or panicky – is important. Thinking like this is upsetting, tiring and affects how you live. The good news is that it's possible to help change things to get your life back into balance.

Noticing extreme and unhelpful thinking

The next step is to practise ways of **noticing** anxious thinking. Watching for times when you have extreme and unhelpful thoughts is the first and most important step in beginning to change how you think. Once you can notice these patterns in your thinking you can step back and choose to make changes.

Here are some examples of how extreme thinking may affect how you feel and what you do.

Example: John's unhelpful thinking

John is going shopping. As he gets ready to leave home, he suddenly realises that he can't find his wallet (= **people and events around me**). He jumps immediately to the worst conclusion that his wallet and credit cards were stolen the last time he was out (= **altered thinking**). This makes him feel very anxious and panicky. What he thinks has affected how he feels (= **altered feelings**). He begins to notice a sick feeling in his stomach. He also feels quite sweaty and clammy and has a tense feeling in his head (= **altered physical symptoms**). He immediately contacts his credit card agency and bank to cancel his cards (= **altered behaviour**).

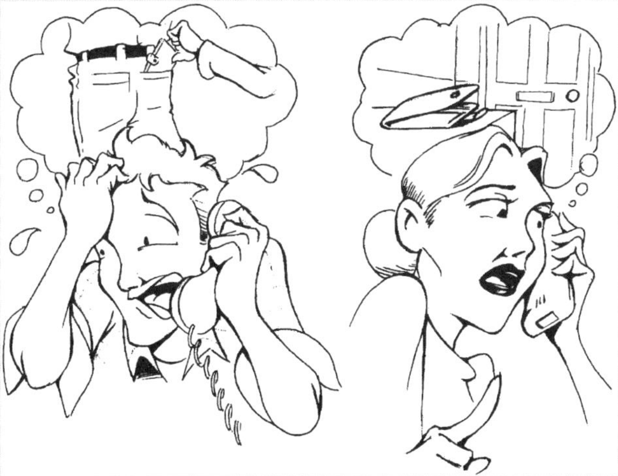

John then phones his friend Anne to tell her what has happened. She is sympathetic and encourages John to try to remember where he last saw the wallet. Anne suggests that he looks around the house to see if he can find it. John thanks her and is pleased that he called because he feels a little better as a result. He promises to phone Anne back that evening to let her know if he finds the wallet.

Later that day he finds the wallet in his coat pocket. He realises he had forgotten he put it there yesterday. He then tried to avoid seeing or talking to Anne because he is worried that she will think he is 'a right fool'. He doesn't phone her back that evening to let her know he has found the wallet.

John's Five Areas thought review of a time when he felt worse

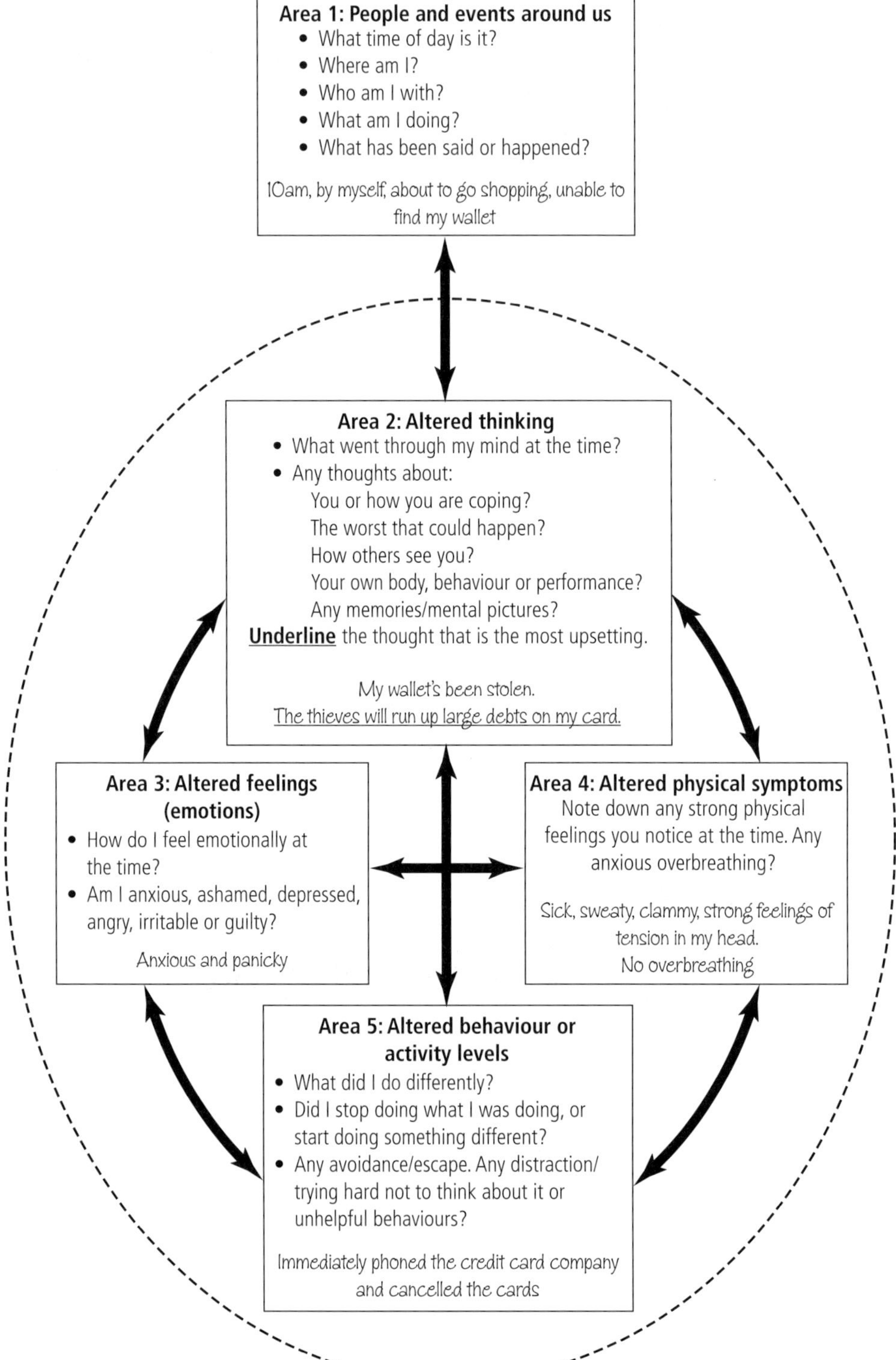

Example: Anne fears a broken friendship

Anne is wondering why John has not phoned her back. He had promised he would. Why hasn't he? (= **people and events around me**). Anne begins to worry that she may have sounded irritable towards him. The fact is that John has phoned her before in similar situations when he can't find something important. She knows that he usually finds the lost thing after having a proper search. She worries that she might not have been supportive enough.

Anne blames herself for upsetting John and not being a good friend (= **altered thinking**). She feels guilty (= **altered feelings**). That night Anne can't relax (= **altered physical symptoms**) and lies awake worrying that she has upset John and harmed their friendship. She decides not to phone him for a few days (= **altered behaviour**) because she is not sure how he might react if she really has upset him. Perhaps he will break off their friendship?

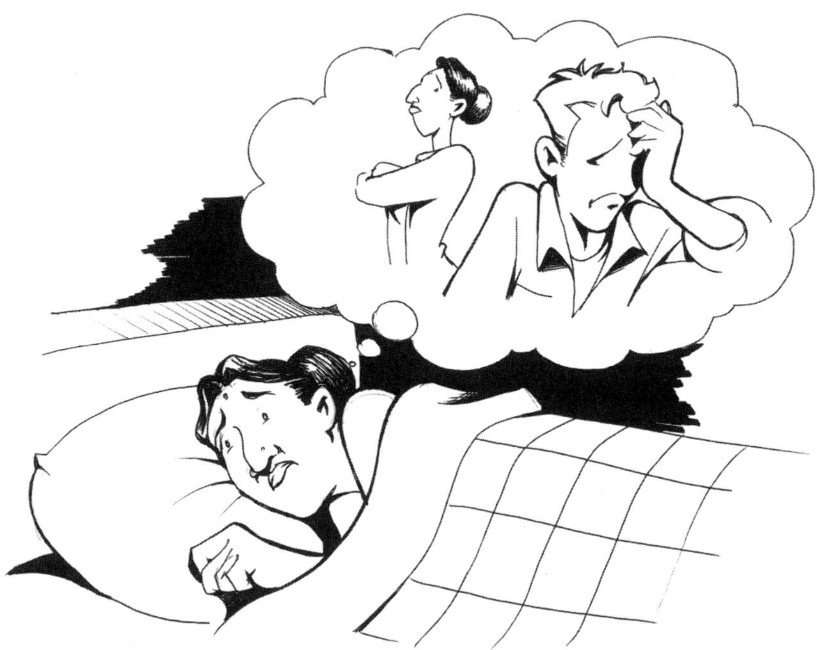

Anne's Five Areas thought review of a time when she felt worse

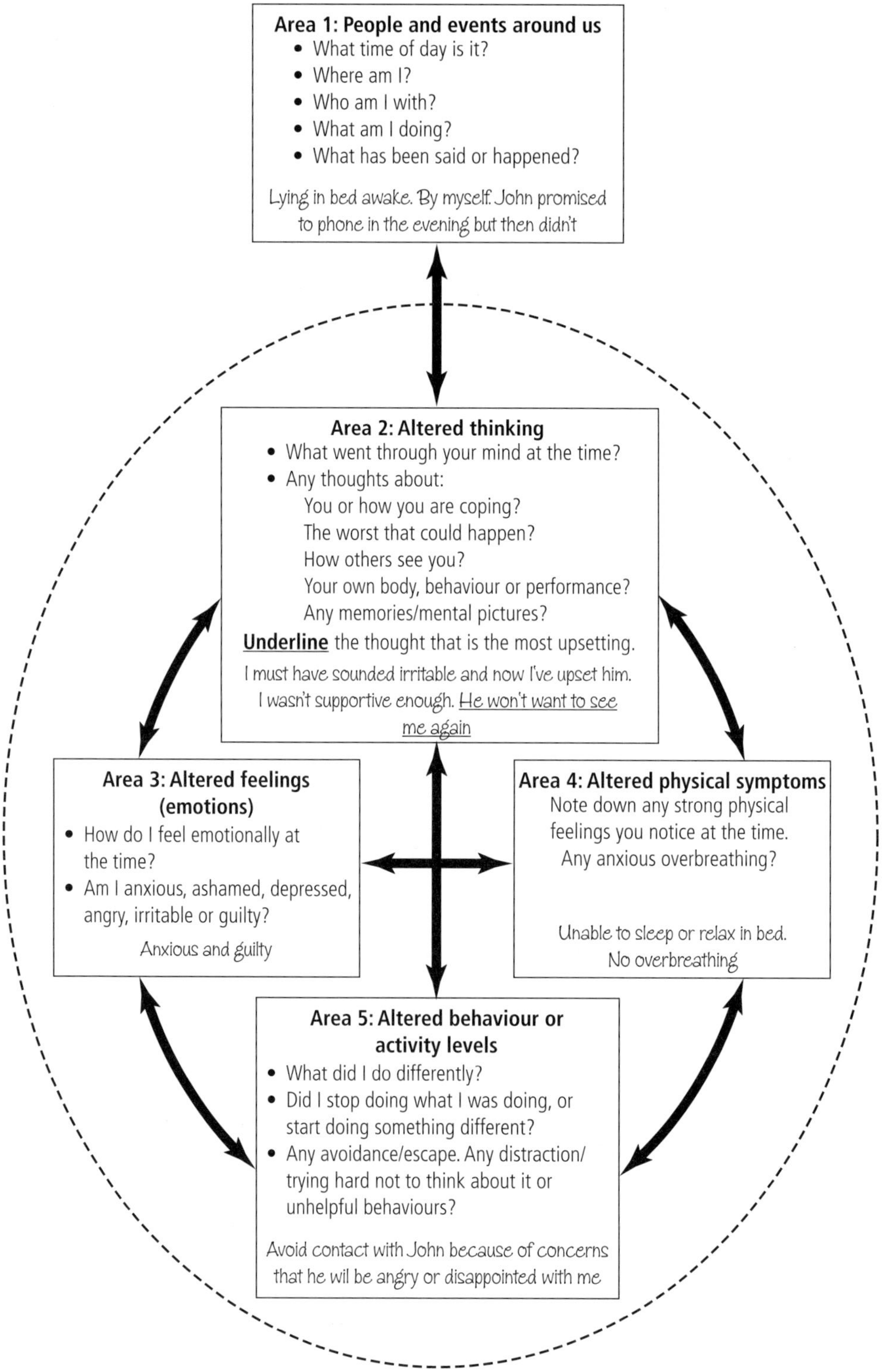

Area 1: People and events around us

- What time of day is it?
- Where am I?
- Who am I with?
- What am I doing?
- What has been said or happened?

Lying in bed awake. By myself. John promised to phone in the evening but then didn't

Area 2: Altered thinking

- What went through your mind at the time?
- Any thoughts about:
  - You or how you are coping?
  - The worst that could happen?
  - How others see you?
  - Your own body, behaviour or performance?
  - Any memories/mental pictures?

Underline the thought that is the most upsetting.

I must have sounded irritable and now I've upset him. I wasn't supportive enough. He won't want to see me again

Area 3: Altered feelings (emotions)

- How do I feel emotionally at the time?
- Am I anxious, ashamed, depressed, angry, irritable or guilty?

Anxious and guilty

Area 4: Altered physical symptoms

Note down any strong physical feelings you notice at the time. Any anxious overbreathing?

Unable to sleep or relax in bed. No overbreathing

Area 5: Altered behaviour or activity levels

- What did I do differently?
- Did I stop doing what I was doing, or start doing something different?
- Any avoidance/escape. Any distraction/trying hard not to think about it or unhelpful behaviours?

Avoid contact with John because of concerns that he wil be angry or disappointed with me

In these two examples, John and Anne's fears (**jumping to the very worst conclusion** and **mind-reading** what the other person thought) led them to feel more anxious. Something that would have taken only a few minutes to sort out on the phone resulted in much worry over the following hours. It also unhelpfully affected how they behaved. In spite of their worries, neither Anne nor John actually did something to check out how the other had reacted. If they had, they would have realised quite how unhelpful and wrong their fears were.

These examples also show that it is not necessarily the events themselves that cause upset, but your **interpretation** of the event. In anxiety and depression, people tend to develop more extreme, negative and unhelpful thinking styles. These thoughts can build up out of all proportion, and unhelpfully affect how you feel and what you do. This can prolong your feelings of distress.

Completing your own thought review

Now let's look in detail at a particular time when you felt worse.

First, try to think yourself back into a situation in the past few days when your mood unhelpfully changed. To begin with **don't choose a time when you have felt very distressed**. Instead, pick an occasion when you were not too upset – and had at least some anxiety/stress or tension symptoms, anger or guilt. Try to be as slow as you can when you think back through the situation, so that you're as accurate as you can be. If you can't think of such a situation, carry on reading. If you can think of one go straight to the task below.

What to do if you find it's hard to even think about the upsetting situation

Sometimes it can feel distressing going back over a time when you have felt worse. That's why it's important to choose a time that didn't make you feel too upset.

The idea here is to make you feel able to change such thoughts and to feel less distressed. Sometimes concerns, worries and fears can feel terrifying and too much to look at all in one go. **So if you feel this way, the key is to practise this approach slowly, with less upsetting thoughts to begin with.**

Start to notice the thoughts that link in with feeling **somewhat or moderately stressed, scared or upset**. Work with these thoughts first, and use the rest of the workbook to practise changing these. You can slowly work up to more upsetting thoughts later when you are feeling more confident.

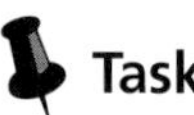 **Task**

Now stop, think and reflect as you go through the five different areas that can be affected. Use the blank Five Areas diagram on page 304 to go through what you noticed in each of the Five Areas.

1. **People and events around you**: Think about the situation.
   - Where were you and what time of the day was it?
   - Who else was there and what was said?
   - What happened?

   Write the answers in Box 1 of the Five Areas diagram.

2. **Altered thinking**:
   - What went through your mind at the time and how did you see yourself?
   - How were you coping (for example, did you think badly of your own self)?
   - What did you think was the worst thing that could happen (were you expecting the worst, that is, catastrophic thinking)?
   - How did you think others saw you (were you mind-reading)?
   - What did you think about your own body and behaviour?
   - Were there any painful memories from the past?
   - Did you think up any images or pictures in your mind (images are another way of thinking and can have a powerful effect on how you feel)?

   Write down any thoughts you notice in Box 2. **Underline** the most upsetting thought.

3. **Altered feelings (emotions)**:
   - Were you feeling anxious, ashamed, depressed, angry or guilty at the time?

   Write these things in Box 3.

4. **Altered physical symptoms**:

   You may have noticed changes in your body when you are angry or anxious, for example:

   - Muscle tension, jitteriness or pain.
   - Rapid heartbeat and breathing; feeling hot, sweaty, clammy.
   - Poor concentration and feelings of low energy, pressure or even pain.

   Write these things in Box 4.

5. **Altered behaviour or activity levels**:

   Was there any:

   - *Reduced activity* – you reduced or stopped doing what you had planned to do.
   - *Avoidance or escape* – you felt anxious and avoided doing something or left without staying to see if the thing you fear really happened.
   - *Unhelpful behaviours* – you tried to block how you felt by acting in ways that backfired in the longer term. For example trying to distract yourself, seek reassurance or drink excessive alcohol or take street drugs.

   Write these things in Box 5.

At the same time, did you also notice that there were other, more helpful, responses that you made?

My Five Areas thought review of a time when I felt worse

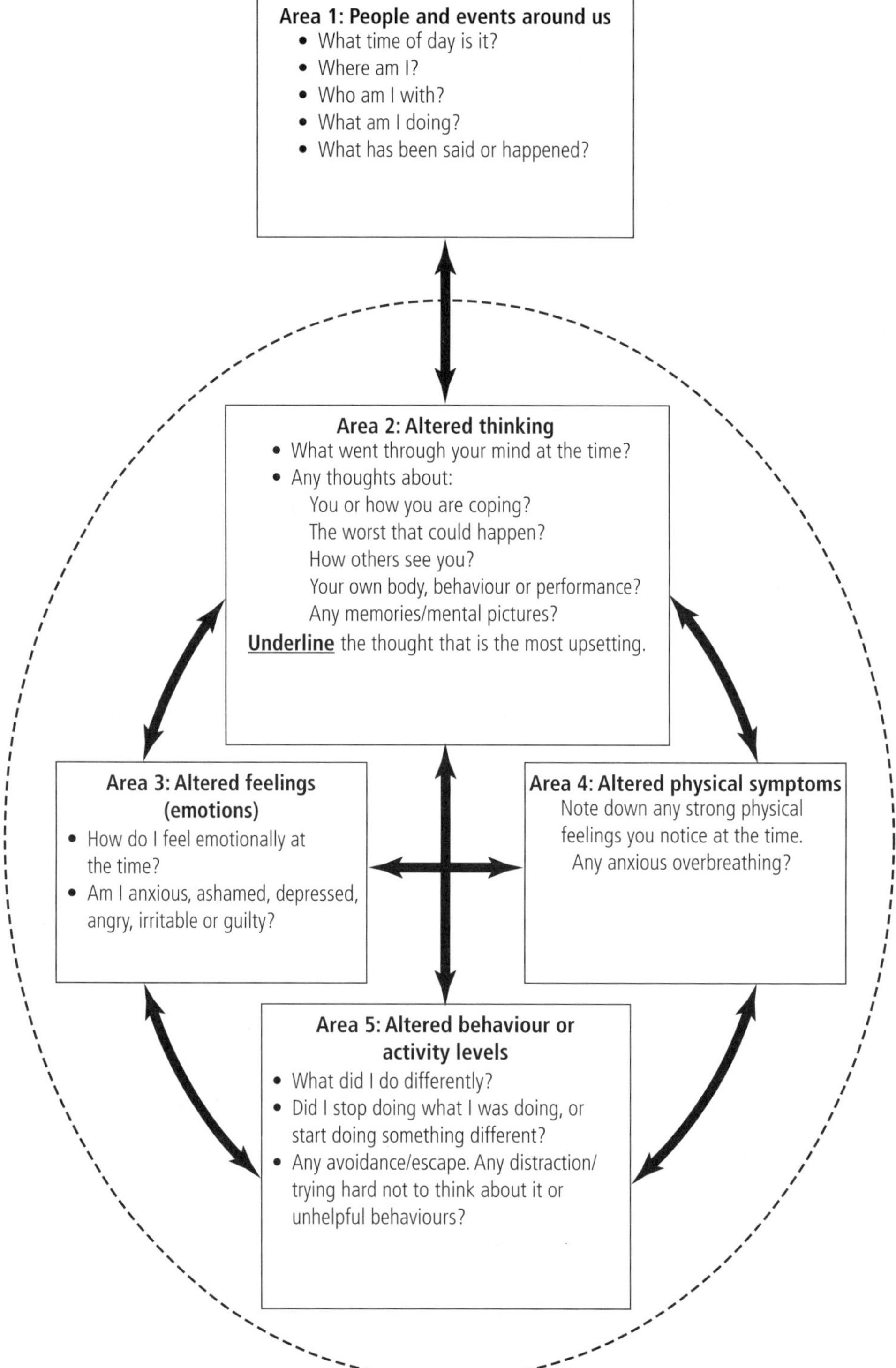

Hopefully, the Five Areas model has shown you that **what you think** about a situation or problem may **affect how you feel** physically and emotionally. It may also alter **what you do** (altered behaviour).

What you think ↔ affects how you feel.

What you think ↔ affects what you do.

Q Does your thought review show this?

Yes ☐ No ☐

There is another blank Five Areas assessment sheet at the end of this workbook. Copy this so you can practise this approach again and again. Doing this is helpful because being aware of these patterns is an important step towards changing things. You can download these for free from **www.fiveareas.com**.

At first, many people find it can be quite hard to notice their unhelpful thinking. By doing the thought review described here you will be able to start noticing this kind of thinking. Over time you'll find that it will become easier and easier to do so. The best way of becoming aware of your thinking is to try to notice the times when your mood unhelpfully alters (for example at times when you feel anxious, irritable, low or panicky), and to then ask 'What is going through my mind right now?'

Remember, everyone has all kinds of thoughts during the day. The thoughts you need to change are those that are:

- *Extreme* – that is, they show one of the unhelpful thinking styles described in the table on page 307.
- *Unhelpful* – that is, they worsen how you feel and/or affect what you do.

Changing extreme and unhelpful thoughts

Sometimes people try to cope with anxiety by trying not to think about it. *Is this a good way of coping?* To see if this works, you can do this practical experiment.

Look at the picture below. Now try as hard as you can to **not think** about the white polar bear for the next 30 seconds.

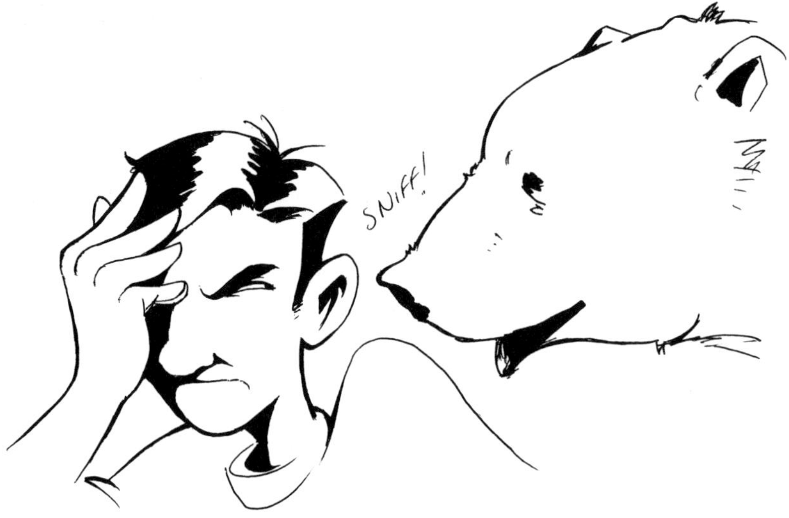

After 30 seconds, think about what happened.

Was it easy not to think about the bear, or did it take a lot of effort? You may have noticed that trying hard not to think about it actually made it worse! Or, you may have made a lot of mental effort trying hard to think about something else such as a *black polar bear*. This is very like anxious worrying. When people try very hard not to worry, it just makes things worse. That is why you need to find new and more effective ways of identifying and then challenging your worrying thoughts.

The following five steps are a **proved way of changing thoughts** that are extreme and unhelpful. You can use as many or as few of the following steps as you need. Just stop when you feel you can move on from the thought.

1. Label the thought as 'just one of those unhelpful thoughts', rather than 'the truth'.
2. Stop, think and reflect – don't get caught up in the thought.
3. Move on – act against it. Don't be put off what you were going to do.
4. Respond by giving yourself a truly caring response.

Try to act like a scientist:

5. Put the thought under a microscope and ask yourself the seven thought challenge questions.

Let's look at each of the steps one at a time.

Step 1: Label the thought as 'just one of those unhelpful thoughts'

When you feel upset, use the list below to tick the unhelpful thinking patterns that are present at that time.

Unhelpful thinking style	Tick if your thought(s) showed this pattern at that time
Am I being my own worst critic? (Biased against yourself)	☐
Am I focusing on the bad in situations? (A negative mental filter)	☐
Am I making negative predictions about the future? (A gloomy view of the future)	☐
Am I jumping to the very worst conclusion? (Catastrophising)	☐
Am I second-guessing that others see me badly without checking if it's actually true? (Mind-reading)	☐
Am I *taking unfair responsibility* for things that aren't really my fault/taking all the blame?	☐
Am I using unhelpful *must/should/ought/got to* statements? (Making extreme statements or setting impossible standards)	☐

Key point

If the thought *doesn't* show one of the unhelpful thinking styles then you should stop here. Choose another time when you feel more upset, anxious, panicky, low, angry, ashamed or guilty and complete Step 1 again until you identify a thought that is an unhelpful thinking style. Then move on to Step 2.

Step 2: Stop, think and reflect – don't get caught up in it

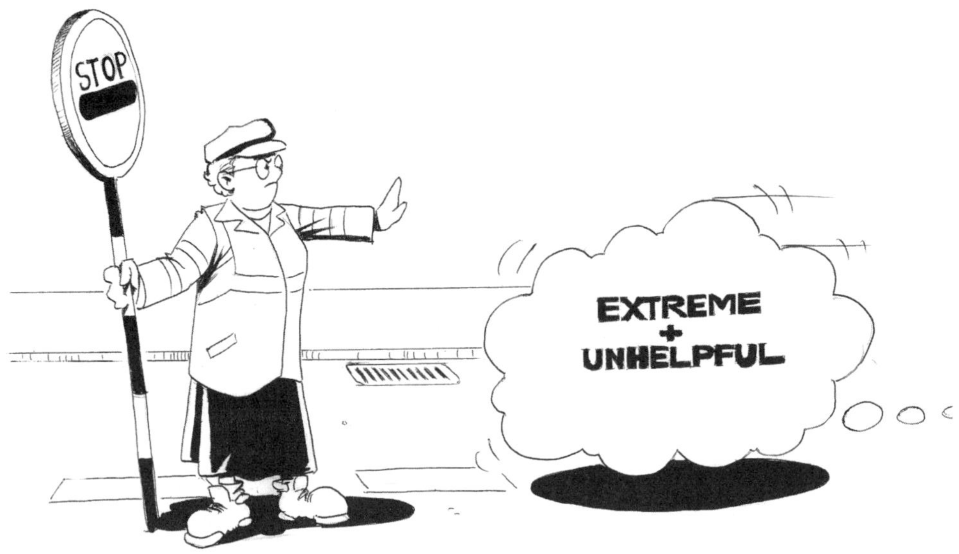

Simply **noticing** that you're having an unhelpful thinking style can be a powerful way of getting rid of it.

- Label the upsetting thought as **just another** of those unhelpful or even silly thoughts. These are just a part of what happens when you are upset. It will go away and lose its power. It's part of distress – it's not the true picture. You could say to the thought: 'I've found you out – I'm not going to play that game again!'
- You might notice that you often have the same types of thoughts. It can be helpful to label them in groups: 'Oh here come my "work's a nightmare thoughts"', or 'Here are my "I can't cope thoughts"' – giving a name can reduce the power of the thoughts over you.
- Allow the thought to **just be**. Don't let yourself get caught up in it. Don't bother trying to challenge the thought, or argue yourself out of it. Like a celebrity, such thoughts love attention. But remember, they are just not worth it. Take a mental step back from the thought as if observing it from a distance. Move your mind on to other more helpful things – for example, the future, or recent things you have done well. One thing that may help is to choose a tune you know well and enjoy, and hum it quietly (e.g. *Jingle bells*). Perhaps even better is to busy yourself with doing the task in hand.

Example: Coping with junk email

If you have a computer and an email address, you will be getting junk email. When you receive junk email, you can either spend a long time getting upset by it, reading it and deleting it, or just accept that it's part of life – like extreme thoughts that are unwanted. So how you cope with the junk mail (rage, anger, focus on the unfairness) and how much time you spend on it will vary. You might just note the email subject header and decide you don't fancy a degree, Viagra, or to import £10 million from the wife of a dead general and simply delete it. Or you may spend time reading it, replying to it and then learning that by replying you end up with even more junk mail.

Unhelpful thoughts are like junk email – the more you try to reply to them the worse they can get. So you need to spot them, decide not to spend too much of your time and life on them and delete them from your mind. And then don't go fishing around in the recycle bin!

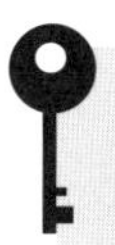

Key point

Making a sensible choice to let a thought 'just be' is different from times of anxiety or panic, when you also might try to distract yourself away from thoughts. But in distraction you try very hard not to think about the situation – such as how you are feeling in your mind or your body. The activity is driven by desperation, worry and fear. This is very different from the active and planned choice to let the worrying and scary thoughts just be.

Worry doesn't actually sort out problems. Extreme, scary thoughts are usually not true – the worst don't happen most of the time. Another unhelpful thing about trying to distract yourself is that it's a very short-term fix to a longer term problem and uses up loads of energy. Letting thoughts be or labelling thoughts is a conscious decision not to spend time going down that fearful route again. You are in control and making the choice – rather than being pushed around and bullied by your fears.

Step 3: Move on – act against it. Don't be put off from what you were going to do

Unhelpful thinking worsens how you feel and alters what you do in a negative way. The thought may push you into:

- Reducing your activity levels by not doing as much as before. This leads to a loss of pleasure, achievement or closeness to others. In the longer term it will restrict your life and undermine your confidence.
- Avoiding or escaping from a situation that seems scary or too difficult by hurrying away or speeding up.
- Distracting yourself *mentally* by trying hard not to think about how you feel (for example, desperately saying 'I'm alright' again and again or focusing on the lines on the floor) or through actions such as biting your lip or digging your nails into your hand, etc.
- Starting to respond in ways that backfire and make you feel worse. For example seeking reassurance again and again from others, or pushing others away, losing your temper for no good reason or having too much alcohol to block how you feel.

Make an **active choice** not to allow these things to happen again. This often means acting against the thought. Choose to react helpfully rather than unhelpfully. Choose not to be bullied into changing what you do by the thought.

To stand up to your unhelpful thoughts try these dos and don'ts.

Do:

- **Keep doing** what you planned to do anyway. Stay active.
- **Face your fears**. Act against thoughts that tell you that things are too scary and you should avoid them. By taking a step-by-step approach you can overcome these fears. See the *Facing fears and overcoming avoidance* workbook.
- **Experiment**: If an extreme and unhelpful thought says don't do something – do it. If a thought says you won't enjoy going to that party, go and see if you do or don't.

Don't:

- Get pushed into not doing things by the thoughts.
- Let fear rule your life.
- Block how you feel with drink or even drugs or by seeking reassurance.
- Accept a life where you cope by avoiding and escaping.

Step 4: Respond by giving yourself a truly caring response

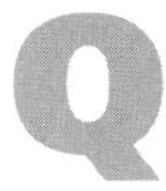

What would someone who wholly and totally loved me say?

When you feel stressed or scared, you may often be very critical of yourself. People can say things to themselves that they would never say to someone they cared for. If a friend was troubled by a thought or worry, you would offer words of advice to soothe and encourage them. Imagine you have the best friend in the world. Someone who is totally on your side, totally loving and is totally caring. What words of advice and encouragement would they say to you? Write their caring advice here:

Think about this – choose to apply their words in your own situation. Trust what they say. Allow that trust to wash over you and take away the troubling thoughts.

You might choose a close friend or relative – or perhaps a famous person from literature, or, if you have a religious faith, someone from your scriptures. Whoever you choose you need to be aware that the response will be unconditionally positive, caring and supportive. Once you have written it down also speak it out loud (when you're alone!), and say the words to yourself again and again in a compassionate voice.

Example: Anne's caring thoughts

Anne chooses her Gran. She thinks back to what she would have said – words of support and love: 'You know we all love you Anne. People often worry about things when they feel upset. You're just worrying. Just let it be. If John is upset you'll find out in good time but – you know what – I bet he isn't. You listened to him when he needed it. He's probably just found his wallet and is embarrassed to say. It's not worth upsetting yourself about. You can always have a chat with him tomorrow. He'll be pleased to see you – just you see.'

Step 5: Put the thought under a microscope and ask yourself the seven thought challenge questions

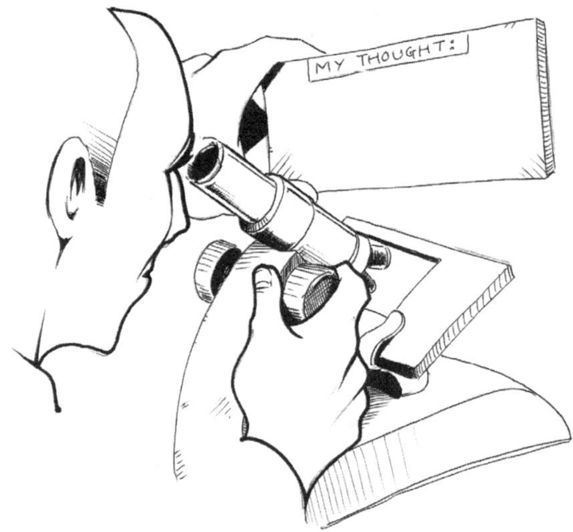

Our upsetting thoughts are often incorrect and untrue. Pretend you're a scientist, and look at the thought in a logical way.

The questions you need to ask are:

- What would I tell a friend who said the same thing?
- Am I basing this on how I feel rather than on the facts?
- What would other people say?

- Am I looking at the whole picture?
- Does it really matter so much?
- What would I say about this in six months time from now?
- Do I apply one set of standards to myself and another to others?

The Worry Box

One problem with worry is that you go over and over the same ground again and again. Sometimes worries can con you into thinking that worry is a great solution to sorting out problems. In fact problem solving (as described in the *How to start fixing problems and finding solutions (practical problem solving)* workbook) is the best way of solving problems. Worry doesn't involve problem solving at all. It just involves going over things again, and again, and again.

A helpful solution is to create several *Worry* boxes for your own use. Use something like a shoe box or similar. If you are artistic then paint it up so it looks nice. In each box place a copy of the following two workbooks:

- *How to start fixing problems and finding solutions (practical problem solving)*
- *Noticing and changing anxious thinking* (the workbook you are reading – but finish reading it first!)

Also put a pen, and some blank paper in the boxes. Position these by your bed, by your desk and by the settee. Then, when a worrying thought pops into mind you can note it down, together with a **time and date** when you are able to deal with it properly and put it in the box. That way there's no need to worry about it just now (useful if, for example, you are trying to get to sleep).

When you get to that time and day (e.g. Thursday 10 a.m.) sit down and work out a solution, or choose to let the worry just be. If it's a focused, practical problem, use the *How to start fixing problems and finding solutions (practical problem solving)* workbook (if it's something you need to sort out). If it doesn't involve something that needs to be fixed, then the *Noticing and changing anxious thinking* workbook is the one for you.

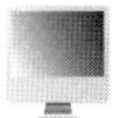

You can download some Worry slips/notes for free from **www.fiveareas.com**. Or create your own (just write My Worry on a piece of paper, and the time and date you'll tackle it).

Taking what works for you

When you use the approaches described above in this workbook, you'll probably find that some responses work better for you than others. Build the ones that work for you into your own reaction for when you notice upsetting thoughts. Remember, practising really helps.

Also **discussing** your thoughts, fears and concerns with others can sometimes help you see them **differently**. And so they will no longer seem upsetting. Finally, make a summary of all the information you have about the upsetting thought.

Example: Sam changes her mind

Sam often finds herself mind-reading that others at work find her boring – but she decides that she will not withdraw and be quiet. So that lunch time, instead of sitting in the corner of the room as usual, she deliberately sits with her colleagues. She asks them how their weekend went. Everyone is friendly and they have a nice talk. Several people ask what she has done over the weekend – and say that they like her hair cut.

These actions help Sam change her perspective and feel less anxious. By choosing to go and talk, Sam realises some important things:

- First, people were friendly.
- Second, she did quite enjoy it – especially when she was complimented on her hair.

Summary

In this workbook you have learned to:

- Recognise patterns of anxious thinking that worsen how you feel.
- Respond to upsetting thoughts in ways that help.
- Change this sort of thinking so it's less upsetting.

The approach you have worked through will work for any extreme and unhelpful anxious thoughts that make you feel worse. By labelling, stepping back from and challenging these thoughts, you will begin to change the way you see yourself, the way things are right now and how they will be in the future.

What have I learnt from this workbook?

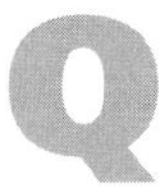
What do I want to try *next*?

Putting into practice what you have learned

You will find blank thought practice worksheets at the end of this workbook. Please copy them if you need more. You can also download more sheets for free from the Five Areas website (**www.fiveareas.com**).

Getting the most from the thought worksheets

- Practise using the approach whenever you notice your mood is changing unhelpfully. In this way, you'll find it easier to notice and change your extreme and unhelpful thinking.
- Try to challenge your unhelpful thoughts **as soon as possible** after you notice your mood change.
- With practice, you'll find that you can work out what are the most helpful parts of this workbook for you and use them to help you in everyday life.

Getting more help

The separate resource *The Worry Box* provides more hints and tips for dealing with worrying thinking. This book and free downloadable colour worksheets to help you spot unhelpful thinking, label unhelpful thoughts and work on changing them are available from **www.fiveareas.com**.

Acknowledgement

Thank you to Catriona Kent for the Coping with junk mail example. The concept of the 'compassionate mind' response was developed by Professor Paul Gilbert, among others.

My notes

Practice sheets

My Five Areas thought review of a time when I felt worse

Write in your thoughts in all Five Areas.

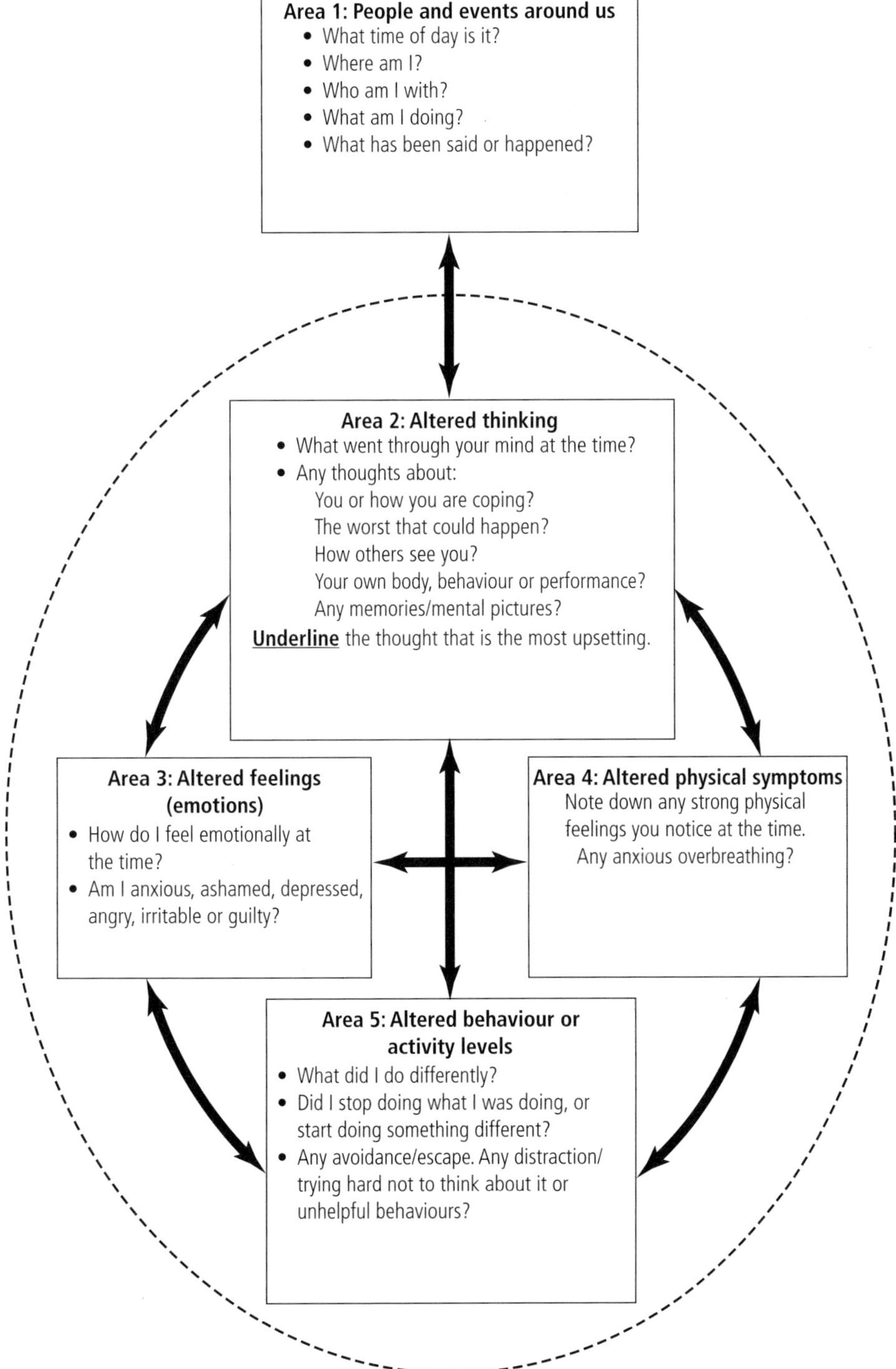

The key steps of the thought review

Use the responses below that work for you.

1. **Label the thought** as 'just one of those unhelpful thoughts'.
    - Am I being my own worst critic? (Bias against yourself)
    - Am I focusing on the bad in situations? (A negative mental filter)
    - Am I making negative predictions about the future? (A gloomy view of the future)
    - Am I jumping to the very worst conclusion? (Catastrophising)
    - Am I second-guessing that others see me badly without checking if it's actually true? (Mind-reading)
    - Am I taking unfair responsibility for things that aren't really my fault/taking all the blame?
    - Am I using unhelpful must/should/ought/got to statements? (Making extreme statements or setting impossible standards).
2. **Stop, think and reflect**: Don't get caught up in the thought.
3. **Move on**:
    - Don't be put off from what you were going to do.
    - Keep active. Face your fears.
    - Keep to your plan. Respond helpfully.
    - Don't be bullied. Act against the upsetting thought and see what happens.
4. Respond by giving yourself a **truly caring response** – for example what would someone who loved you wholly and totally say?

5. Ask the thought these seven hard questions:
   - What would I tell a friend who said the same thing?
   - Am I basing this on how I feel rather than on the facts?
   - What would other people say?
   - Am I looking at the whole picture?
   - Does it really matter so much?
   - What would I say about this looking back six months from the future?
   - Do I apply one set of standards to myself and another to others?

Another helpful option is to write down your worries – and state a time and date when you will tackle them. This will help you to solve the problem you face, or deal with your worries. Creating your own Worry Box can help you practise this approach.

Remember: It will take time and practise to build your confidence in using this approach. A downloadable, credit-card sized version of this summary is available free of charge from the Five Areas website (**www.fiveareas.com**). You can also get free Worry strips from the website.

Overcoming Anxiety, Stress and Panic
A Five Areas Approach

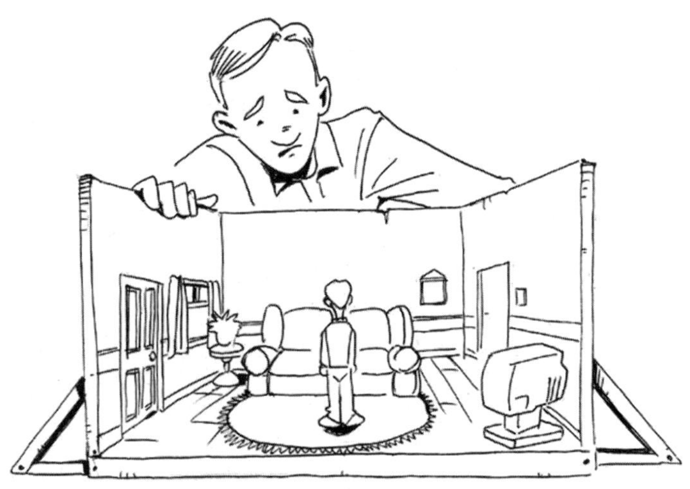

Understanding and overcoming feelings of depersonalisation

www.livinglifetothefull.com
www.fiveareas.com

Dr Chris Williams

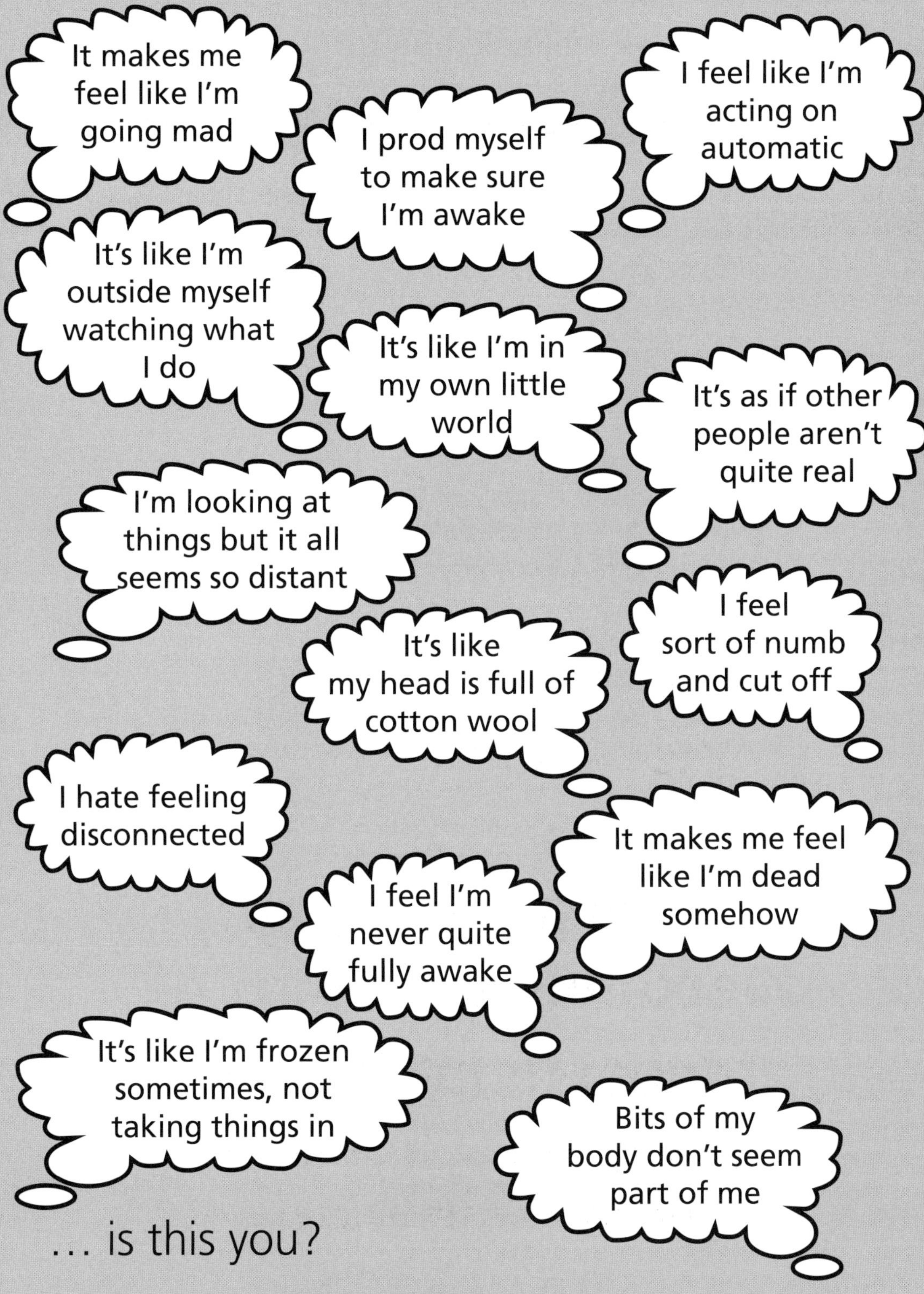
It makes me feel like I'm going mad
I prod myself to make sure I'm awake
I feel like I'm acting on automatic
It's like I'm outside myself watching what I do
It's like I'm in my own little world
It's as if other people aren't quite real
I'm looking at things but it all seems so distant
It's like my head is full of cotton wool
I feel sort of numb and cut off
I hate feeling disconnected
I feel I'm never quite fully awake
It makes me feel like I'm dead somehow
It's like I'm frozen sometimes, not taking things in
Bits of my body don't seem part of me

… is this you?

If so … this **workbook is for you**

This workbook will help you to:

- Understand what depersonalisation means.
- Understand how depersonalisation can affect you.
- Find out what causes depersonalisation.
- Identify some things you can do to try to improve your own problems of depersonalisation.

What is depersonalisation?

Many people who have problems with anxiety or depression can feel mentally cut-off from themselves from time to time. This feeling is called *depersonalisation*, and it can last for hours or days or longer. It can be hard to describe exactly what depersonalisation feels like. You may get a *fuzzy-headed, spaced-out* sort of feeling. You know that you are fully awake, yet you feel distanced from yourself, your body or your feelings. You may feel like you are a robot acting on automatic.

Sometimes people feel like they are an observer – looking at everything from a distance. The outside world may seem like a giant theatre set. You know it's there but it seems far away and not quite right. This feeling that things around you may not seem completely real – is called *derealisation*. These feelings can be very unsettling.

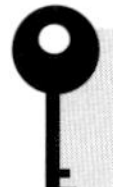

Key point

Depersonalisation and derealisation often start suddenly, and just as suddenly stop.

This workbook uses the term depersonalisation to describe all the above experiences. The important thing to remember is that your senses (sight, touch, smell, etc) all continue to work quite normally – but how you perceive or view what is going on changes from the usual way you do this.

Q Do you sometimes feel that you are cut-off from the outside world – not quite connecting?

Yes ☐ No ☐ Sometimes ☐

Q Do you feel that you seem cut-off from other people – so they say things but you feel like it isn't really going in?

Yes ☐ No ☐ Sometimes ☐

Q Do you feel that you seem cut-off from your bodily senses such as touch, hearing or seeing things – or as if part of your body is not feeling things properly?

Yes ☐ No ☐ Sometimes ☐

Q Do you feel cut-off from you and your own thinking or emotions so that you are almost like an observer looking at yourself or as if your emotions are deadened?

Yes ☐ No ☐ Sometimes ☐

Q Is this an unpleasant feeling you would prefer to have stop?

Yes ☐ No ☐ Sometimes ☐

If you answered 'Yes' or 'Sometimes' to any of the questions above, depersonalisation is a problem for you.

The next step is to discover what might be causing you to feel this way.

What causes depersonalisation to happen?

Depersonalisation is quite a common condition. It happens to many people, as part of daily life. Researchers think depersonalisation happens when a part of your brain, which controls your emotions, is switched on or off. What switches that part of your brain on or off is usually something that makes you stressed. This may be something within your own body or something else from outside. Studies seem to show that about 40 per cent of people have this built-in switch, which makes them prone to depersonalisation.

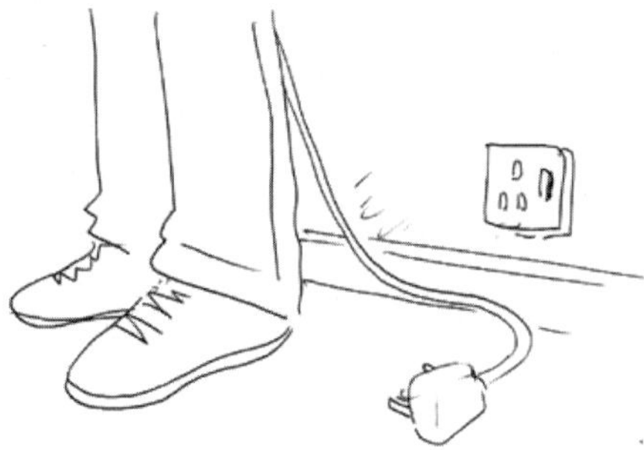

There are several different triggers that can set off the built-in switch and lead to depersonalisation. Here are the most common ones.

1. **High levels of anxiety or panic.** High levels of emotion including anxiety or panic can cause depersonalisation. Anxiety may be the result of everyday stresses, or the depersonalisation itself may make you more anxious. For example, during an attack of depersonalisation people sometimes feel they are going mad or losing their mind.
2. **Anxious overbreathing (hyperventilation).** Usually, when you become fearful, your body reacts to this. Your heart rate and rate of breathing both increase. If you are hyperventilating, you take *rapid short breaths* through the mouth. Even though you are getting more than enough oxygen into your blood supply, you feel some unpleasant but harmless physical symptoms. This can include depersonalisation, as well as other symptoms such as dizziness, blurred vision, a dry mouth, and a feeling of tightness in your chest.
3. **High levels of depression.** When people are depressed, they feel excessively down and few if any things can cheer them up. People who have problems with anxiety or panic often also have depression. Physical symptoms of depression include feeling low in energy, not feeling like eating and sleeping poorly. Depersonalisation often happens to people with high levels of depression.
4. **Tiredness** is also a common cause of depersonalisation.
5. **Drinking too much alcohol or using street drugs.** Some stimulant street drugs can switch on depersonalisation. Also, you may get into a cycle of using alcohol to block the feelings to some extent. The problem with over-drinking is that it can quite quickly become unhelpful and backfire – causing even more problems.

6. **Upsetting memories/flashbacks and other upsetting thoughts.** Sometimes, memories/flashbacks of an upsetting event or trauma in the past can cause people to feel more upset or tense – this can also lead to depersonalisation. Sometimes you may be only dimly aware of the thoughts, but instead you may be more aware of the unpleasant feeling of depersonalisation. If you have unpleasant memories of the past, you should discuss with your doctor whether you need to see a specialist. For example, your doctor may refer you for cognitive behavioural therapy (a kind of talking treatment).

Many physical illnesses can also trigger depersonalisation. For example:

- **Infections** – such as colds/flu/viral infections.
- Undiagnosed or under-treated **high blood pressure** (hypertension).

Depersonalisation and medication

Depersonalisation can sometimes happen **as a side effect of medication**. Many common medications can lead to feelings of depersonalisation. These medicines include those prescribed for both mental and physical health problems, for example anti-depressant medications. If you are taking medication ask your doctor if this is a known side effect.

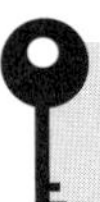

Key point

Are the symptoms a side effect of medication?

Most medications do not cause depersonalisation in most people. But if you have depression or depression and anxiety, it is more likely, on balance, that the cause is the emotional upset. So it's important not to stop the medication without an open discussion with your own doctor about this.

A useful clue that suggests a possible link between taking a medication and having depersonalisation is whether it *started or worsened* after you began to take (or increased the dose of) the particular medication. Also watch to see if the symptoms worsen regularly 30 minutes to two hours after taking the medication.

If you and your doctor jointly agree that medication might be a factor in your depersonalisation you can test this out by:

- Changing to another type of medication that treats the same condition.
- Reducing the dose of the current medication.
- Changing the timing of when you take it (for example, at night-time when you are asleep).
- Having a time off the medication.

These changes can be viewed as an experiment. Record the *severity* and *length of time* you notice the depersonalisation. Do this for one week or so **before** and **after** any change in medication. This will help you make a judgement together about whether the medication is causing your symptoms.

Depersonalisation and epilepsy

A certain type of epilepsy called *temporal lobe epilepsy* can cause symptoms of depersonalisation. Most people think of epileptic fits as causing the person to lose consciousness while shaking their limbs. However, some forms of epilepsy can occur while the person is fully awake and otherwise functioning normally. Temporal lobe epilepsy is one of these examples of so-called *partial* epilepsy. The word 'partial' means that there is a fit but it's not so bad as to cause a loss of consciousness.

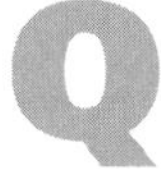

Is depersonalisation being caused by epilepsy?

The following questions ask you about several symptoms that can be present in temporal lobe epilepsy. Please note that if you give a positive response to several of the questions, this only suggests that temporal lobe epilepsy *could be considered*. The questions are not intended to make a diagnosis of epilepsy. If you think you might have epilepsy, you should discuss this with your doctor.

Q Have you ever had a fit or an unexplained loss of consciousness?

Yes ☐ No ☐ Sometimes ☐

Q Do you ever notice strange smells or strange tastes in your mouth that don't seem to have a usual explanation?

Yes ☐ No ☐ Sometimes ☐

Q Do you find that sometimes when you visit a place you know you have gone to before, you don't have any sense of familiarity for it at all?

Yes ☐ No ☐ Sometimes ☐

Q Have you ever experienced the reverse of this – visiting somewhere you know you have never been to, yet the place seems very familiar to you? (so-called *déjà vu*).

Yes ☐ No ☐ Sometimes ☐

If you have answered 'Yes' or 'Sometimes' to any of these questions, you should discuss this with your doctor. He or she may suggest you have some tests to check whether temporal lobe epilepsy is present. If they think you do have epilepsy, they may prescribe some anti-epileptic medication. This can be very effective.

If you suspect that some of the possible factors that can lead to depersonalisation are present, please discuss this with your healthcare practitioner so that you can jointly decide how to approach this problem.

Working out what triggers your feelings of depersonalisation

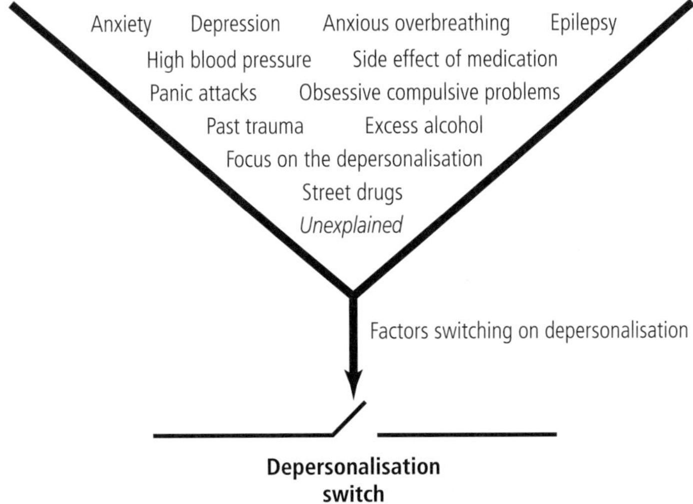

If you can identify the factors that are switching on your depersonalisation, you can try to focus on changing them.

Spotting patterns that affect your depersonalisation

The first thing is to do some research on how you feel. The aim is to play detective and identify any factors that are worsening the situation for you.

Use the Depersonalisation diary at the end of the workbook to record **all the times** when you are feeling depersonalised over the next few days.

Example: Paul rates his depersonalisation

For the past six months Paul has struggled with illness and has been off work. He has started to drink more as well. He feels both depressed and stressed by his lack of a job and by the money worries, which are mounting up.

He has noticed feelings of depersonalisation that last between 10 and 40 minutes. During these times, he feels spaced out and has a 'fuzzy head'. He has seen his doctor to check for possible physical conditions. But he doesn't have epilepsy or high blood pressure. His doctor recommends he keeps a **Depersonalisation diary** and they look through the contents of the last week together.

Things that seem to make Paul's depersonalisation come on are:

- *Stressful pressures or feeling low*: Arguments with his partner Helen increase Paul's stress levels. Especially if they argue and he goes away and feels angry and dwells on things, the symptoms come on even more. They also worsen when he sits fretting about how to pay the bills.
- *Focusing on the depersonalisation symptoms*: Worrying about when it will go away – or whether it will get worse.
- *Sleep and breathing*: He definitely breathes faster and shallower during times of depersonalisation. He notices his shoulders coming up and shoulder tension. He definitely notices the feeling more when he has slept badly.

Things that seem to improve how Paul feels are:

- Becoming less stressed.
- Getting a good night's sleep.
- Trying to relax and enjoy something like a good film.
- Having a bottle of wine.

Together Paul and his doctor agree that though it's tempting to use drink to block how he feels, there are dangers of this backfiring badly.

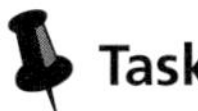

Task

Now keep your own Depersonalisation diary for the next few days. Use the blank diary at the back of this workbook, or copy it. You can download more for free from **www.fiveareas.com**.

How the diary can help you move forwards

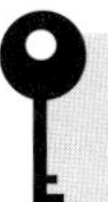

Key point

Use the diary to reflect on how you try to respond – and whether this makes the situation worse. For example, drinking heavily might give some immediate relief, but creates more problems in the longer term.

Write down what you discover about what seems to make your depersonalisation worse or better here:

Q Do I feel worse first thing in the day? (This suggests depression or poor sleep may be a problem.)

Q Do certain situations seem to affect how bad it is? (For example, is it affected by stressful pressures or particular situations such as crowds, or supermarkets?)

Q Do certain emotions seem to affect how bad it is? (For example, is it affected by feeling low, anxious, angry, guilty or ashamed?)

Q Does focusing on or worrying about the depersonalisation symptoms make them worse?

Q Do poor sleep or rapid breathing affect how it feels?

Q Is it affected by exercise?

Q Are there any links to using medication, alcohol or street drugs? (Do you regularly feel worse within a couple of hours of using drink, tablets or street drugs?)

Identify your early warning signs

Use your diary to think back in detail to some of the recent times when you have felt depersonalised. Try to play detective and think about whether there were any early warning signs:

- Either that something which brings on depersonalisation was building up.
- Or that you were beginning to become depersonalised.

Key point

Early warning signs of becoming depersonalised include:

- Altered thinking: getting scared, anxious, panicky or depressed about things.
- Altered emotions/feelings: for example, rising tension, dropping mood, or becoming irritated or angry.
- Altered physical sensations: for example, becoming hot, sweaty, fidgety, noticing more rapid breathing or heart rate, or increased tension.
- Altered behaviour or activity levels: for example, drinking more, prodding yourself to bring yourself back to reality, raising your voice, or avoiding things.

Being able to notice these key early warning signs means you can **do something about it now** before your depersonalisation happens or gets worse. Well done for spotting your early warning signs.

Making changes to avoid depersonalisation

The good news is that you can learn to do something different when you start to feel depersonalised. Use your answers to the questions above to work out what longer-term changes you need to make in your life.

Here are some suggestions that can help:

1. Reduce body tension
   - Drop your shoulders.
   - Continue to take normal sized breaths.
   - If you are tensing up choose to relax your arms or legs.
2. Change the focus of your thoughts
   - Choose not to focus on anything that is stressing you out or making you feel annoyed, hurt or angry. Say to yourself 'I'm not taking that path again'. Don't jump to conclusions. Take a long-term view – it won't matter so much in two weeks.

- Then move your mind onto what else is happening right now, or get involved in doing another activity. One thing that may help is to choose a tune you know well and enjoy and hum it quietly (for example, *Jingle bells*). You can find some more hints and tips in the *Noticing and changing anxious thinking* workbook.

3. Do something different.

Try to do something that is interesting, that involves activity (like exercise), or is meaningful for you or simply fun. Do things with others which can also make you feel closer to them.

4. If you tend to overbreathe or are sleeping poorly:

   - **Practice and use breathing control strategies.** The *Overcoming anxious overbreathing (hyperventilation)* workbook can help.
   - Try to work on **improving your sleep** using the *How to get a good night's sleep: overcoming anxiety and sleep problems* workbook.
   - Other things that can help are exercise (see the *Using exercise to overcome stress* workbook) and dealing with problems with alcohol or street drugs (see the *Stress, alcohol and drugs* workbook).

5. **Don't let the depersonalisation take over your life.** You may be avoiding things and putting things off. If so, use the *Facing fears and overcoming avoidance* workbook to tackle avoidance and reclaim your life.
6. If you think you have anxiety, depression and problems such as an obsessive-compulsive disorder, seek advice from your doctor. If they think you have one of these conditions, they will discuss the various treatment options available with you.
7. A national centre of excellence for the treatment of depersonalisation based in London provides a specialist back-up if other treatments are not helping as much as you would like. You can get information about this clinic, which is based at the Institute of Psychiatry (Maudsley Hospital), from your GP.

What about medication and relaxation?

Doctors don't recommend any medication for depersonalisation. It might seem logical to advise doing relaxation techniques for depersonalisation. Especially if you are feeling anxious and stressed, and have noticed this worsens how you feel. But some people with depersonalisation find that trying to relax and focusing on their body and minds during relaxation actually makes them feel worse. If this happens to you, don't use a relaxation approach. Instead, focus on some of the other things you can do from the ones described above. There are lots of things you can do to tackle depersonalisation.

Summary

In this workbook you have learnt:

- What depersonalisation is.
- How depersonalisation can affect you.
- What causes depersonalisation.
- How to identify some things you can do to try to improve your own problems of depersonalisation.

Q What have I learnt from this workbook?

Q What do I want to try *next*?

Putting what you have learned into practice

Write down what you're going to do this week, to put into practice what you have learnt.

My practice plan

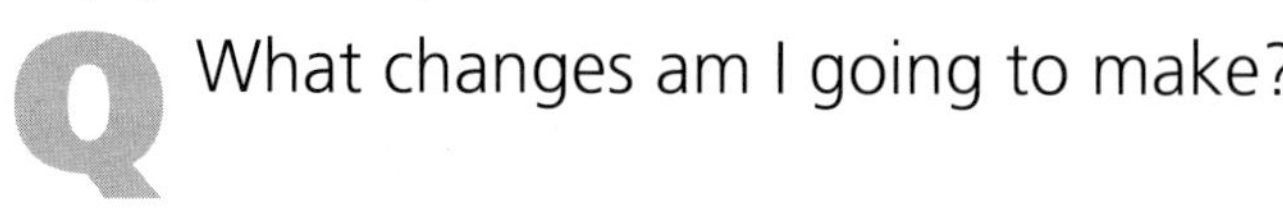

Q What changes am I going to make?

Q When am I going to do it?

Q What problems could arise, and how can I sort these?

Apply the **Questions for effective change** to your plan.

Q Is my planned task one that:

- Will be useful for understanding or changing how I am?

  Yes ☐ No ☐

- Is a specific task so that I will know when I have done it?

  Yes ☐ No ☐

- Is realistic, practical and achievable?

  Yes ☐ No ☐

- Makes clear what I am going to do and when I am going to do it.

  Yes ☐ No ☐

- Is an activity that won't be easily blocked or prevented by practical problems?

  Yes ☐ No ☐

- Will help me to learn useful things even if it doesn't work out perfectly?

  Yes ☐ No ☐

Remember to review your progress in making these changes weekly, and to make sure the changes are practical and achievable.

My notes

Example: My Depersonalisation diary

Date and time	Record your recent sleep, drink/tablets and feelings of pressure that might affect the depresonalisation	People and events around you	My feelings at the time	My thoughts at the time	My physical symptoms at the time	My behaviour at the time
	When things improve also record what you were doing at the time it improved	– Where were you? – Who were you with? – What were you doing? – What was said/ happened?	How did you feel emotionally at the time? – Were you feeling anxious or depressed? – Any other emotions? (irritable, angry, guilty, ashamed?)	Any thoughts about: – Things not being fair? – Being picked on? – Being mocked/ humiliated? – How you are coping? – The worst that could happen? – How others see you? – Your own body, behaviour or performance? – Any memories or mental pictures? – Any really upsetting thoughts or images at the back of your mind you'd rather not consider?	Note down any strong physical symptoms you noticed at the time, e.g. tension, rapid heartbeat, breaking out in a sweat, breathing faster, feeling shaky	– What did you do differently? – What did you say differently – and how did you say it? – Did you stop doing what you were doing, or start doing something different? – Are you avoiding things because of how you feel? Please note down if you were overbreathing at the time (shallow, rapid breaths)

Overcoming Anxiety, Stress and Panic
A Five Areas Approach

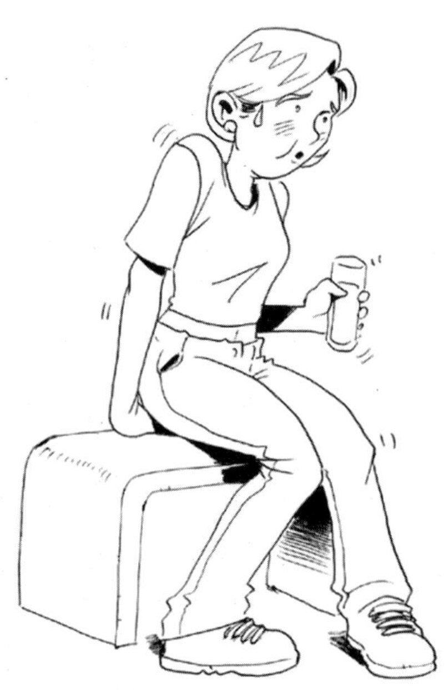

Overcoming anxious, overbreathing (hyperventilation)

www.livinglifetothefull.com
www.fiveareas.com

Dr Chris Williams

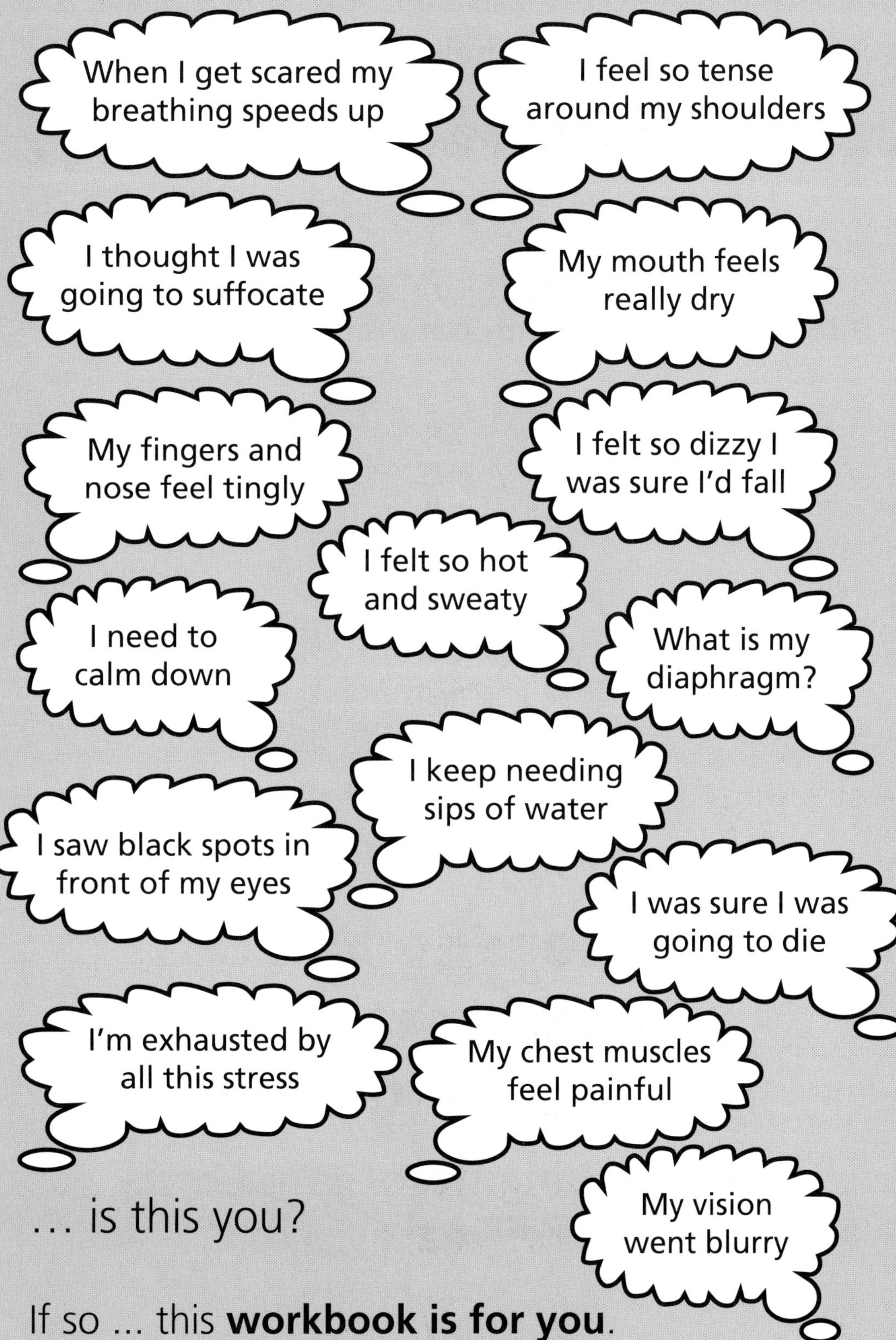

… is this you?

If so … this **workbook is for you**.

This workbook will help you to:

- Discover what anxious overbreathing (hyperventilation) is.
- Understand how breathing like this can affect you.
- Identify some things you can do to control and overcome anxious overbreathing.

Bodily changes during panic and high anxiety

Think about a time when you have had a sudden shock. Perhaps you stepped into the road when a car was coming and didn't realise till you heard the car horn. Did your heart beat a lot faster and did you start to breathe a lot faster too? What makes this happen is the fight or flight adrenaline response.

So blood is pumped faster round your body so that your muscles are ready to react. Then you can try to defend yourself from any potential danger or run away from it. This is very useful when the danger is real.

But your body reacts to frightening thoughts just as it would to a physical danger. The fight or flight adrenaline response will cause your heart rate and breathing both to speed up. There may be other physical responses such as feeling sweaty or restless and tense. Sometimes rapid breathing continues long enough to turn into anxious overbreathing. This is also known as *hyperventilation*.

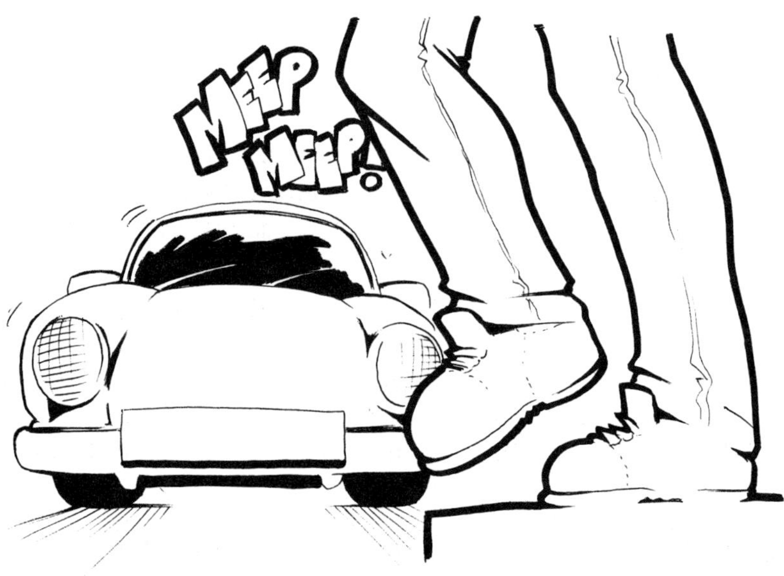

How do your physical changes and catastrophic fears relate to each other?

The fight or flight adrenaline response makes you pay particular attention to any potential dangers around you. But it becomes a problem when you feel scared about things that aren't really that dangerous. For example, you may be scared of going shopping, or riding on a bus. Neither of these are threatening like possibly being hit by a car.

Every person with panic focuses on dangers that are especially scary for them. For example, anxious overbreathing and a tight chest can strengthen fears that 'I'm suffocating'. Likewise a very rapid heart rate or chest pain in panic may support fears that 'I'm having a heart attack'. Feelings of dizziness and blurred vision caused by overbreathing can strengthen fears that 'I am about to faint/collapse' or that 'I'm having a stroke'.

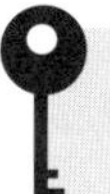

Key point

It is important to recognise that although these feelings are unpleasant, **they are not harmful.**

What is anxious overbreathing?

It is helpful to know the difference between *sudden-onset hyperventilation* (so-called *acute hyperventilation*), which occurs during panic, and the problem of *longer-term hyperventilation* (*chronic hyperventilation*), which is a 'bad habit' of breathing fast.

- When you have **acute hyperventilation**, you breathe faster with the upper part of your chest. You take *rapid short breaths* through the mouth. So even though you are getting more than enough oxygen into your body, you may begin to notice unpleasant but harmless physical symptoms. You may feel breathless and dizzy with blurred vision and a dry mouth. This can lead to a tight feeling in your chest. You may also have tingling at the tip of your nose, your feet, the tips of your fingers or in your hands. Overbreathing can occasionally cause muscle spasms in the hands or face. Finally, it can make you feel dizzy or fuzzy-headed. You may feel 'spaced out', distanced, or strangely disconnected from things.
- If you have **chronic hyperventilation**, you get similar **but milder** symptoms. For example, slight dizziness, occasionally blurred vision, a dry

mouth, and also some tightness in the chest. Again, it can make you feel dizzy or fuzzy-headed so that you feel 'spaced out' and disconnected from things. You may feel short of breath on occasion when anxious, even if you are not exercising. Finally, it can cause you problems with sleep and make you feel tired all the time. Again, it is important to recognise that although these feelings are unpleasant, **they are not harmful**.

Q If you overbreathe, which symptoms do you notice?

- Not getting enough air into your body?

Yes ☐ No ☐ Sometimes ☐

- A dry mouth?

Yes ☐ No ☐ Sometimes ☐

- Blurred vision?

Yes ☐ No ☐ Sometimes ☐

- Tightness in your chest or shortness of breath?

Yes ☐ No ☐ Sometimes ☐

- Tingling in the nose, mouth, fingers or hands?

Yes ☐ No ☐ Sometimes ☐

- Feeling jelly-legged or faint/dizzy?

Yes ☐ No ☐ Sometimes ☐

- A strange fuzzy-headed/disconnected feeling where everything seems to go quite distant?

Yes ☐ No ☐ Sometimes ☐

What causes these symptoms?

In normal breathing, you breathe in oxygen from the air and breathe out a gas called carbon dioxide. When you breathe more rapidly than usual, you breathe out greater amounts of carbon dioxide than you should. It is the reduced amount of carbon dioxide in your body that causes the bodily symptoms seen in hyperventilation. You can slow down your body's loss of carbon dioxide and even reverse this situation by slowing your breathing. This helps you re-capture some of the carbon dioxide so that you quickly begin to feel better again. To do this, you need to close your mouth and take slow, normal-sized breaths.

Most adults take between 12 and 20 breaths a minute. Adults who practise relaxed breathing can reduce this down to six to ten slow deep breaths a minute. In contrast, in hyperventilation, rapid shallow breaths occur at a rate of 20 to 30+ breaths per minute. Interestingly, **people overbreathing like this often describe feeling out of breath**. Have you noticed this happening to you?

If you think you have had an attack of anxious overbreathing for the first time, it is important to discuss this with your doctor. There are many mental health problems that cause panic with anxious overbreathing. For example, depression, anxiety and panic attacks.

Like anxious overbreathing, some physical health problems can also cause you to breather faster. For example:

- Lung problems such as asthma or long-term chest problems such as emphysema (this condition is common in smokers).
- Chest infections (pneumonias).
- Heart problems – which can cause you to feel short of breath when lying down, or cause you to wake up in the early morning feeling short of breath.
- Undiagnosed or under-treated diabetes – when the sugar levels in your body are too high. This can make you overbreathe.

If you think you have a physical condition that's causing you to overbreathe, talk to your doctor. He or she can advise you on whether you may need some tests to check this out or if you need any treatment.

If the cause of your overbreathing is not a physical one, you can do some active things to overcome anxious overbreathing.

Spotting patterns that affect your overbreathing

The first thing is to do some research on how you feel. The aim is to play detective and identify any factors that are causing you to overbreathe.

Use the Anxiety diary at the end of the workbook to record **all the times** when you overbreathe over the next few weeks.

Example: Harvinder records his hyperventilation

Harvinder has been having attacks of anxious overbreathing whenever he goes shopping in large supermarkets. He starts to feel anxious and breathes faster even before he gets to the shops. He records his breathing rate before going shopping, and it is about 22 breaths a minute (increased above his normal resting rate of 18). He notes that he needs to keep an eye on this, and that he might have chronic hyperventilation.

Today, as Harvinder walks to the shop, he begins to worry about what might happen, and his breathing rate increases even more. He starts to feel more anxious and sweaty and his heart speeds up. As he enters the shop he starts to walk even faster, and grips the handle of the shopping trolley for support. He fears that he will collapse and suffocate, and his heart rate and breathing shoot up. His heart rate increases to over 100 beats a minute (normal for him is up to 70 or so), and his breathing increases to 30 breaths a minute. He starts to feel dizzy, with a dry mouth. His head feels like it is swimming and he feels ill. He decides to leave.

Things that seem to make Harvinder's hyperventilation and panic come on are:

- Being in the shop.
- *Stressful pressures or feeling low*: He also notices as he keeps his diary that he is more likely to overbreathe when he feels under pressure generally. For example, he had a previous panic attack when he was travelling to see his boss about a possible return to work.
- *Focusing on the panicky symptoms*: He realises that when he starts getting anxious he starts to scan his body to see how he feels. By noticing and becoming hyper-aware of being sweaty and dizzy, he feels worse and worse.
- *Sleep*: He definitely notices the feeling more when he has slept badly.

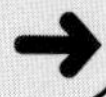

Things that seem to improve how he feels are:

- Being less stressed generally.
- Getting a good night's sleep.
- Slowing down his breathing and walking speed.

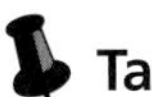 **Task**

Now start keeping your own Anxiety diary for the next few days. Use the blank diary at the back of this workbook, or copy it. You can download more for free from **www.fiveareas.com**.

How the diary can help you move forwards

Write down what you discover that makes your overbreathing worse or better.

Q My patterns during the day (do I feel worse first thing in the day)? (This suggests depression or poor sleep may be a problem.)

Q Do certain situations seem to affect how bad it is? (For example, is it affected by stressful pressures or particular situations such as crowds, or supermarkets?)

Q Do certain emotions seem to affect how bad it is? (For example, is it affected by feeling low, anxious, angry, guilty or ashamed?)

Q Does focusing on or worrying about the hyperventilation symptoms make them worse?

Q Do poor sleep or rapid breathing affect how I feel?

Q Is the overbreathing affected by exercise?

Q Are there any links to using medication, alcohol or street drugs? (Do I regularly feel worse within a couple of hours of using drink, tablets or street drugs?)

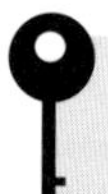

Key point

Use the diary to help identify any factors that make you feel worse. Go through step by step what happens as overbreathing takes hold of you.

Identify your early warning signs

Use your diary to think back in detail to some of the recent times when you have hyperventilated. Try to play detective and think about whether there were any early warning signs:

- Either something was building up and then brought on the overbreathing
- Or you were beginning to start hyperventilating.

Early warning signs of hyperventilation include:

- Altered thinking: getting scared, anxious, panicky or depressed about things.
- Altered emotions/feelings: for example, rising tension, dropping mood, or becoming irritated or angry.
- Altered physical symptoms: for example, becoming hot, sweaty, fidgety, noticing more rapid breathing or heart rate, or increased tension.
- Altered behaviour or activity levels: for example walking faster, misusing asthma inhalers or becoming increasingly restless.

Being able to notice these key early warning signs means you can **do something about it now before your overbreathing becomes worse**. Well done for spotting your early warning signs.

Making changes

Overcoming acute (sudden-onset) hyperventilation

Use your answers to the questions above to work out what longer-term changes you need to make in your life. The good news is that you can learn to do something different when you start to overbreathe.

First, slow down your breathing by taking slower, deeper breaths. At the same time try to:

- Drop your shoulders.
- If you are tensing up choose to relax your arms or legs.
- **Close your mouth**. It is not possible to hyperventilate for long through your nose. If you have a cold this can get quite messy!
- **As before, slow down your breathing rate**. Take slower, normal-sized breaths. This is the reverse of the shallow, rapid breaths that are part of the problem in hyperventilation.

Two handy hints:

- *Count as you breathe*. Count slowly 1, 2, and 3 as you breathe in. Say each number after about a second's interval. Then breathe out again counting 1, 2, and 3. This will help you to slow your breathing down to about seven or eight breaths a minute. Remember to take normal-sized breaths. If this is difficult at first start with deeper breaths and then reduce the size of your breath to normal over a few minutes by using the counting technique.

- *Imagine you are in a peaceful, calm place*. Choose somewhere you would like to visit or a place where you have happy memories of past holidays – perhaps near the sea, watching the waves lapping up and down on the shore. Try to link your breathing to the relaxed movement of the waves. Again aim to slow your breathing down.

These two techniques will help you to stop overbreathing. You should follow this up with longer-term practice of the exercises described later to re-gain a healthy breathing pattern.

Other things you can do to help

- **Change the focus of your thoughts**: choose not to focus on anything that is stressing you or making you feel annoyed, hurt or angry. Move your mind away from how scared or ill you feel. Say to yourself 'I'm not taking that path again'. Don't jump to conclusions. Take a long-term view – it won't matter so much in two weeks. One thing that may help is to choose a tune you know well and enjoy, and hum it quietly (for example, *Jingle bells*).
- **Do something different**: Move your mind onto what else is happening right now, or get involved in doing another activity. You can find some more hints and tips on how to do this in the *Noticing and changing anxious thinking* workbook. Doing things with others can also make you feel closer to them and change your focus.
- If you are sleeping badly, try to work on **improving your sleep** using the *How to get a good night's sleep: overcoming anxiety and sleep problems* workbook.
- Other things that can often help are using exercise (see the *Using exercise to overcome stress* workbook) and dealing with problems with alcohol or street drugs (see the *Stress, alcohol and drugs* workbook).
- **Don't let the overbreathing take over your life**. You may be avoiding things and putting things off. If so, use the *Facing fears and overcoming avoidance* workbook to help you tackle avoidance.
- If you think you have anxiety, depression and problems such as an obsessive-compulsive disorder, seek advice from your doctor. If they think you have one of these conditions, they will discuss the various treatment options available with you.

- If you notice a fuzzy-headed, disconnected feeling when you overbreathe, you may be having an episode of depersonalisation. You can find out more about this condition in the *Understanding and overcoming feelings of depersonalisation* workbook.

Overcoming chronic (longer-term) hyperventilation

The key to overcoming problems of longer-term hyperventilation is to develop more relaxed breathing habits. In hyperventilation, you forget the normal slower, deep-breathing pattern as a result of anxiety. The result is that you take shallow breaths using just the upper part of your chest, like in anxious hyperventilation. This again breathes off carbon dioxide, and can make you feel unwell.

Experiment:

When you notice overbreathing, push on the muscles between the ribs of the upper chest as you breathe in. The muscles will feel tense and tight. Pressing them is painful as a result.

The good news is that it is possible to re-learn healthy habits of breathing. It's helpful first to understand how relaxed breathing – so called diaphragmatic breathing – happens.

Relaxed, healthy breathing uses a muscle called the *diaphragm*. This muscle separates your chest from your abdomen/tummy. By using the diaphragm, you can do relaxed, slow, deep breathing.

To feel where your diaphragm is, try to blow up a balloon, or breathe out against a closed mouth. You will notice tension at the top of your abdomen, just below the chest. Push gently just below the ribs and you will feel a large muscle. This is your diaphragm.

Re-learning how to breathe in a relaxed way using your diaphragm

There are several exercises that can work well to help your body get back into the habit of breathing using the diaphragm. You are then more likely to breathe like this throughout the rest of the day, without even having to think about it. Try to persevere. It will take about a week or more of exercise before you notice a reasonable change.

Exercises to re-gain your diaphragmatic breathing pattern

Note: If you have chest problems such as emphysema, heart disease or chronic obstructive airways disease, please discuss the exercises with your doctor before practising them.

Exercise 1

1. Breathe in through your nose while counting silently to three. Then:

   - Record the length of time you can breathe out saying:

     s → (that is, sssssssssssssssssss).

     Do this once or twice first so that you can use it as a baseline to compare with later as you practise the other exercises. Concentrate on slowly controlling how you breathe out using your diaphragm. You will feel this muscle working as you breathe out. Aim to slowly increase the time you take as you breathe out. An average would be 12–15 seconds with no discomfort and not too much tension.

   - Breathe out slowly as a sigh:

     h →

     Again, feel your diaphragm gently tense as you breathe out.

2. Breathe in gently through your nose over a silent, slow count of three.

   Then pause for a count of three.

3. Finally, breathe out slowly through your mouth for a count of three. Try this for only one or two breaths and relax. Settle your breathing before trying again to avoid any dizziness.

   As you practise this, gently extend the time spent breathing out to a count of three, four and so on. Try to reach 8–10. Try to make sure you do this in a relaxed way. The aim is to re-gain a relaxed rhythm to your breathing.

Exercise 2

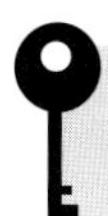

Key point

Be aware of any tension in, or too much movement of, your shoulders. This is a useful marker of the shallow rapid breathing that is a problem in anxiety. As you breathe out, relax your shoulders and be aware of any tension in your neck or your upper back and shoulders.

Do: watch for visible movement of your diaphragm. Remember, the diaphragm is situated just below your ribs at the top of your abdomen.

Don't raise your shoulders – let them drop down in a relaxed way instead. You want to reduce any anxious overbreathing and tension in the upper part of your chest.

Breathe in gently then breathe out slowly through your mouth. Correct any shoulder movement. Also, reduce any anxious overbreathing with the upper part of your chest.

Exercise 3

Produce the sounds drawn below. By doing so you are controlling the rate of air being breathed out by using the diaphragm.

ssssssssS

sSSSSssss

sssssSSSSSsssss

sssssSSSSSsssssSSSSSsssss

shshshshsh

shshshshsh

sh------sh------sh

sh------sh------sh------sh------sh------sh------sh

Try each exercise on three separate occasions first. Then practise doing them several times each day. You don't have to do all the exercises in one sitting though.

These exercises teach you how to create gentle variations in the depth of your breathing – and help you focus on healthy breathing using your diaphragm. With regular practice over several weeks, you should notice that your breathing develops a more natural and relaxed rhythm.

Getting further help

Sometimes advice from a specialist who teaches effective breathing control is helpful. Discuss this with your healthcare practitioner if you are interested in learning more about this approach. Also, singing or playing a wind or brass instrument is a very good way to practise breathing diaphragmatically, while doing something enjoyable. So if you think you could do this, see if there is a choir or a group around that you could join, for instruction and fun.

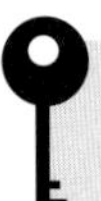

Key point

This workbook has particularly focused on some practical things you can do to overcome hyperventilation. But it is likely that overbreathing is only one of the ways that anxiety is affecting you. Anxiety affects your thinking. It also alters your emotions, causes physical symptoms and alters your behaviour and activity levels. It can also affect how you react to others, and the different situations, places and people that you deal with. You may therefore need to also work on overcoming problems in each of these areas.

Summary

In this workbook you have:

- Discovered what anxious overbreathing (hyperventilation) is.
- Understood how breathing like this can affect you.
- Identified some things you can do to control and overcome anxious overbreathing.

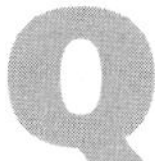
What have I learnt from this workbook?

What do I want to try *next*?

Putting into practice what you have learned

Plan to identify and then change the things that make you prone to anxious overbreathing.

Write down what you're going to do this week, to put into practice what you have learnt.

My practice plan

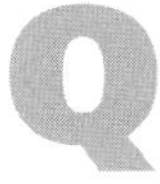
What changes am I going to make?

When am I going to do it?

What problems could arise, and how can I sort these?

Apply the **Questions for effective change** to your plan.

Is my planned task one that:

- Will be useful for understanding or changing how I am?

  Yes ☐ No ☐

- Is a specific task so that I will know when I have done it?

  Yes ☐ No ☐

- Is realistic, practical and achievable?

  Yes ☐ No ☐

- Makes clear what I am going to do and when I am going to do it.

  Yes ☐ No ☐

- Is an activity that won't be easily blocked or prevented by practical problems?

  Yes ☐ No ☐

- Will help me to learn useful things even if it doesn't work out perfectly?

  Yes ☐ No ☐

  Remember to review your progress in making these changes weekly, and to make sure the changes are practical and achievable.

- Do the diaphragmatic breathing exercises regularly – even when you feel your breathing is now fine.

View this as an action plan that can help you to change how you are and tackle your problems of overbreathing.

Acknowledgements

Thank you to Sandra Kinnear for helpful comments and suggested exercises to promote diaphragmatic breathing.

My notes

My Anxiety diary

Date and time	Record your recent sleep /drink/tablets and feelings of pressure leading up to the anxiety	People and events leading up to feeling worse	My feelings at the time	My thoughts at the time	My physical symptoms at the time	My altered behaviour at the time
	When things improve also record what you were doing at the time they improved	– Where were you? – Who were you with? – What were you doing? – What was said/happened?	How were you feeling at the time? – Were you feeling anxious and panicky? – Any low mood? – Any other feelings (irritability, anger, guilt, shame)?	Any thoughts about: – Things not being fair? – Being picked on? – Being mocked/humiliated? – How you are coping? – The worst that could happen? – How others see you? – Your own body, behaviour or performance? – Any memories or mental pictures?	Note down any strong physical symptoms you noticed at the time, e.g. tension, rapid heartbeat, breaking out in a sweat, breathing faster, feeling shaky.	– What did you do differently? – What did you say differently – and how did you say it? – Did you stop doing what you were doing, or start doing something different? – Are you avoiding things because of how you feel? Please note down if you were overbreathing at the time (shallow, rapid breaths)